Towards Better Pract

Library of General Practice Vol 9

Editorial Board

Chairman
John Fry OBE MD FRCS FRCGP

James D.E. Knox MD FRCP FRCGP
M. Keith Thompson FRCGP DObstRCOG
John H. Walker MD FFCM FRCGP DPH
Ian M. Stanley MD ChB MRCP FRCGP

Vol. 1 **Hypertension** *F. Tudor Hart*
Vol. 2 **The First Year of Life** *G. Curtis Fenkins & R. Newton*
Vol. 3 **Rheumatology in General Practice** *M. Rogers & N. Williams*
Vol. 4 **Renal Medicine and Urology** *D. Brooks & N. Mallick*
Vol. 5 **The Use of Computers in General Practice** *F. Preece*
Vol. 6 **Sexual Medicine** *G.R. Freedman*
Vol. 7 **The Care of the Elderly in General Practice** *M. Keith Thompson*
Vol. 8 **Respiratory Disorders** *T. Fry, R. White & M. Whitfield*

Forthcoming volumes in the series

Ischaemic Heart Disease *P. Dootson & D. Rowlands*
Anxiety and Depression *F. Grabinar & M. Lader*
The GP and the Laboratory *R.A.M. Oliver, W.R.G. Thomas & T.R. Tickner*
ENT Disorders *G. Hickish*
Gastrointestinal Disorders *D.A. Coffman, L.J. Chalstrey & G. Smith-Laing*
Gynaecology and Obstetrics in General Practice *F.W. Eddy & F.D. Owen*

The **Library of General Practice** is a series of books for GPs about medical problems as they present in the community. The editorial board is chaired by John Fry, OBE, MD, FRCS, FRCGP — himself a GP and also an experienced author and researcher and a member of the Council of the Royal College of General Practitioners.

Each volume deals with an important aspect of general practice, written by a GP well-known for his work in the field, often in association with a leading specialist in the field.

Practice Libary said of the first volume in the series:

'... if they are all equally good, this series will be a very important contribution to the educational material available in the general practice field ...'

If you would like further information on any of the titles, or details on how to order them, please write to:

Library of General Practice, Sales Promotion Department, Churchill Livingstone, Robert Stevenson House, 1-3 Baxter's Place, Leith Walk, EDINBURGH, EH1 3AF, UK

Towards Better Practice

9

Peter Martin
MB BS FRCGP
General Practitioner, Basildon, Essex; Associate Regional Adviser for North East Thames

Alistair J. Moulds
MB ChB MRCGP
General Practitioner, Basildon, Essex

Patrick J.C. Kerrigan
MB ChB MRCGP
General Practitioner, Basildon, Essex; Consultant Medical Editor to *Pulse*

CHURCHILL LIVINGSTONE
EDINBURGH LONDON MELBOURNE AND NEW YORK 1985

CHURCHILL LIVINGSTONE
Medical Division of Longman Group Limited

Distributed in the United States of America by Churchill Livingstone Inc., 1560 Broadway, New York, N.Y. 10036, and by associated companies, branches and representatives throughout the world.

© Longman Group Limited 1985

All rights reserved. No part of this publication may be reproduced, stored in a retrieval system, or transmitted in any form or by any means, electronic, mechanical, photocopying, recording or otherwise, without the prior permission of the publishers (Churchill Livingstone, Robert Stevenson House, 1-3 Baxter's Place, Leith Walk, Edinburgh EH1 3AF)

First published 1985

ISBN 0 443 028605
ISSN 0263-9742

British Library Cataloguing in Publication Data
Martin, Peter
 Towards better practice. — (Library of general practice, ISSN 0263-9742; v. 9)
 1. Family medicine — Great Britain
 I. Title   II. Moulds, A.J.
 III. Kerrigan, Patrick J.C.   IV. Series
 362.1'72'0941   R729.5.G4

Library of Congress Cataloging in Publication Data
Martin, P.B.
 Towards better practice.

 (Library of general practice; vol. 9)Includes index.
 1. Family medicine — Practice. I. Moulds, A.J.
II. Kerrigan, Patrick J.C.   III. Title.   IV. Series:
Library of general practice; v. 9.   [DNLM: 1. Family
Practice.   W1   L102C   v. 9 / W 89 M926t]
R729.5.G4M68   1984   610   84–14977

Printed in Singapore by Selector Printing Co (Pte) Ltd

Preface

'It is unfortunate, considering that enthusiasm moves the world, that so few enthusiasts can be trusted to speak the truth'

Arthur James Balfour

Being enthusiastic about our jobs as general practitioners we have spent a lot of time thinking and arguing about what we do. Having expended so much energy we decided to write this book, both to clarify our own ideas and to help others to clarify theirs.

While many of our ideas are original, others have been shamelessly borrowed or stolen whenever they have seemed to fit in with our philosophy of care. We have no scruples about such intellectual plagiarism, but would like to acknowledge gratefully the great debt we owe to others.

We think we have arrived at some truths, though we are keenly aware that other practitioners may have very different ideas which are equally valid. In spite of the fact that so much of our preferred method of practice is open to argument, we have presented our case didactically. We hope this will aid critical appraisal.

Deciding how to practise is altogether easier than putting the ideas into effect. What we describe we have achieved to a variable extent — like everyone, we have our individual strengths and weaknesses. We think we know which way our practice is going, but it will take us some time and much more effort to get there. Perhaps slow progress is a blessing in disguise, as it allows for changes of mind both on the route and the destination!

Basildon,	A.J.M.
Essex	P.M.
1985	P.J.C.K.

Acknowledgement

We would like to thank our partners and the many people who work with us in our health centre for their support and stimulation. Most of all we should like to thank them for being so much fun to work with and for making general practice such an exciting and enjoyable place to be.

Contents

Section 1 — Setting the Scene	1
Introduction	3
The effects of the NHS	5
Section 2 — Keeping the Patients Well and Happy	17
Introduction	19
The way forward	21
Providing personal care	23
Giving appropriate care	32
Preventing disease	49
Being accessible	64
Promoting comfort and convenience	71
Section 3 — Keeping the Doctor Happy	77
Introduction	79
Choosing a practice	81
Getting on with partners	85
Maintaining standards	92
Consulting comfortably	108
Managing workload	119
Maximising income	127
Remaining friendly with colleagues	138
Remembering your family and yourself	142
Section 4 — Keeping the Team Harmonious	147
Introduction	149
The team is dead, long live the team	150
Employing responsibly	156
Making the most of receptionists	160
Creating a role for secretaries and practice managers	166

Getting the best out of nurses	171
Cooperating with health visitors	177
All abroad the 'S.S. Caritas'	180

Section 5 — Nuts and Bolts — 185

Introduction	187
Practice premises	188
The appointment system	191
Receptionist training	193
Practice nurses	197
Preparing a job description	202
Record keeping	207
The age-sex register	220
Immunisation systems	223
Repeat prescribing systems	227
Computers	231
Patient education	233
Preparing a practice protocol	237
Practical audit	241
Learning about the consultation	247
Becoming a training practice	250
Medical politics	253
Index	257

Section 1
Setting the scene

Introduction

The style, content and organisation of the work of general practitioners in the UK has few parallels in other countries. Although British GPs are self-employed, independent contractors, their labour is virtually monopolised by the state-run medical service. The bulk of their remuneration is from the National Health Service and is made up of a large 'salaried' element of basic allowances and a crudely work-sensitive element of capitation fees and fees for items of service. Being an independent contractor gives the GP a legitimate tax saving status. State support: including the doctor's pay, a generous occupation pension, 70 percent of staff costs, funds for building surgeries; protects GPs from normal commercial risks and absolves them from the majority of business problems and costs. Thus GPs get the best of both worlds.

In exchange for state support, the GP is obliged to provide all necessary primary medical care for the patients on his or her list, all day and every day. The patients' and the doctors' concepts of what constitutes necessary primary care vary enormously from area to area and from practice to practice. In theory, patients have unrestricted access to the service, with no financial barriers, and can present the doctor with any problem they consider appropriate. Superficially this would appear to be a recipe for a high level of demand and, indeed, some doctors do seem to believe that their patients make unreasonable demands of them. In fact, annual consultation rates and prescription rates per person are much lower here than in most other European countries and, by any objective comparisons, British GPs do not have to see as much of their patients as do their continental colleagues.

Present patterns of practice are the result of an evolutionary process which has moulded the health services and the attitudes of both doctors and patients. Until the advent of the NHS, general practitioners were entrepreneurs who worked single-handed or in very small groups, offering a highly personalised service to their patients. Practice was, on the whole, very competitive and, having little in the way of therapeutic weapons, personality, bedside manner and service were the only wares the GP had to offer to attract and retain his customers. Doctor behaviour was ordered by the need to compete and to please. Patient expectations were in turn moulded and reinforced by this behaviour. The result was a pattern of practice that encouraged both home visiting and unnecessary repeat visits to the surgery and which was very treatment/prescription orientated. Paying patients, then as now, had to be seen to be getting 'good value' for their money — such value seldom being represented by simple advice on the self-management of minor illnesses, particularly as such advice might help the patient to avoid seeing and, hence, paying the doctor in the future!

These behaviour patterns still condition the working habits of many doctors today. Of course, doctors rationalise their behaviour and will produce scientific or ethical reasons to explain patterns of practice which, in reality, owe more to the need to provide the doctor with a reasonable living and to enhance his or her status than to any objective realisation that they represent the best form of practice available. For many doctors this behaviour is neither cynical nor conscious but is rather due to an inability, or at any rate a great reluctance, to stand back and analyse their work with some scientific detachment.

All doctors need to convince themselves as well as others that their main motivating force is patient welfare and that all other considerations are secondary. Financial survival is therefore not normally an acceptable reason for doing things a certain way. Thus, the doctor who needs to carry out a lot of home visits, because it is the tradition in a highly competitive area, will talk about how home visiting improves the doctor–patient relationship and enables more information to be gleaned about social conditions. Another, who has pared home visiting to an absolute minimum, will point out that patients get swifter and better treatment in the surgery, while ignoring the problems that may face the patient in coming to the surgery.

The effects of the NHS

In between the two World Wars most general practice in Britain was carried out on a fee for item of service basis, though a scheme was introduced where working men were able to get treatment under a 'panel' system. Some GPs also ran small private clubs where patients could get any necessary attention in exchange for a small regular subscription.

In 1948 every person in the country became entitled to register with the general practitioner of their choice. The doctor was paid on a capitation basis, and so income was almost entirely dependent on the practice list size and was quite unrelated to the quality or quantity of the medical care provided. In fact, because almost any service incurs some expense, the more the doctor did for the patients the less money there was to put in the bank at the end of the day.

General practitioners were in the position of having to fulfil patient expectations which had largely been formed by the behaviour of their doctors in pre-NHS days. Much of this medical activity was unnecessary and illogical, though this was, and is still, no worse than in any other country. So, in the early days of the NHS and in many areas of the country to this day, practice remained very competitive, probably because of fossilised attitudes rather than compelling economic need. The size of the practice list was viewed as being of paramount importance, being equated with financial stability and professional success. In order to attract and to keep patients, practitioners generally did their best not to offend them in any way by declining to fulfil any of their demands.

On the other hand, the public were particularly lucky in the UK to have inherited such a well-established general practitioner system. By tradition, specialists only saw patients referred to them by GPs, while the practice in other countries where family doctoring was not held in high esteem was by self-referral. This allowed the best, and almost unique, feature of British general practice to develop, namely the long-term relationship between the patient, the family and their family doctor.

When the NHS was introduced, in the face of considerable opposition from the profession, many GPs felt resentful about being forced to join, even though the coercion was financial and not legislative. During the 1950s morale among GPs gradually fell because of low pay, low status and high workloads. Already undercapitalised, there was no incentive to invest in good premises, staff or equipment, and the bulk of doctors worked in relative professional isolation from their own homes with only the help of their wives. The capitation system did not encourage the provision of a good service and, by the early 1960s, morale was so low that mass resignation by GPs became a distinct possibility. This threat and a favourable political climate wrung a new deal from the government of the day which became known as 'The GP's charter' (1965–66).

This altered the system of payment of GPs and provided material resources for good practice separate from the doctor's income, and an income for the doctor less dependent on the size of the practice list. It encouraged doctors to practise in groups, to improve and invest in their premises, to employ ancillary staff, and to work with the help of other professionals such as nurses and health visitors. The underlying assumption was that changes in practice organisation could help to maximise the effectiveness of primary medical care and benefit both patients and doctors. It also resulted in the building of suitably sited health centres to encourage doctors to practise in areas where they were most needed.

At about the same time the level of academic interest and activity within general practice increased dramatically, and a number of GPs began to explore and to write about practice problems. Morale improved, and corporate pride and enthusiasm for their work developed rapidly among GPs. The financial and academic stimuli combined to produce many changes in the methods and conditions of work in practice. This process of development is still going on, though two of the biggest organisational changes that resulted, namely the growth of appointment systems and the decline in home visiting, are unlikely to undergo further dramatic change.

THE PRESENT STATE

Before we move on to look at the problems of present-day general practice, it might be helpful to consider briefly some of the factors influencing workload.

In 1952 in England and Wales there were 17 204 principals in general practice, 43 percent of whom worked single-handed. By 1980 the total was 23 184 and the proportion in single-handed practice had dropped to 14 percent (Fig. 1.1). As the morale and conditions of work have improved, so recruitment to general practice has increased, and in 1982 there were 29 240 GPs in Great Britain with an average list size of 2017. This represents a return to the levels of the 1950s and, if the current trend continues, should reach an average of 1800 by the turn of the century.

List sizes by themselves, however, provide only a very rough guide to workload, and of more significance are the demands made by the patients and how the doctor reacts to them. For instance, the number of consultations per patient per year varies from over 6 in parts of Scotland to about 1.6 in parts of suburban south-east England, with the national average being about 3.5. There are even wider variations in home visiting rates, from 0.1 to 2 per patient per year, even between practices with very similar populations, and of course significant differences in the age (Table 1.1) and class structures of practice populations will also result in a variation in demand, both quantitative and qualitative.

Despite such basic differences and bitter complaints from many GPs of being overworked, it is rare for any of us to spend more than

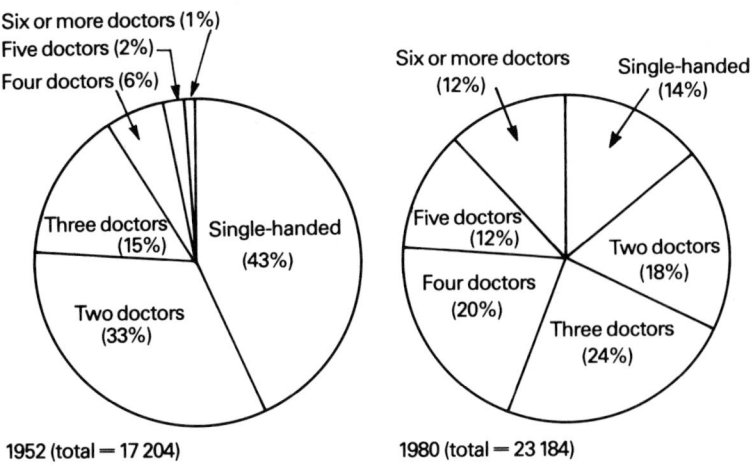

Fig. 1.1 Distribution and number of principals.

Table 1.1 Population distribution (in a practice of 10 000)

Children under 15	2500
15–44	4000
45–64	2000
65–75	1000
Over 75	500

20–30 hours a week face to face with patients; and many doctors manage to hold down a wide variety of extra-practice jobs at the same time. Even if one excludes the effects of delegating work to paramedical staff, marked differences in workload do appear to owe more to the long-term effects of doctor behaviour than to basic differences in the needs of patients. Socio-economic factors do exert profound effects on morbidity, but it is quite easy to find gross differences in perceived workload between practices serving very similar populations. The harassed GP struggling to cope with the practice workload may find it difficult to accept that he or she can significantly alter patient expectations. A little thought, however, should make it clear that most significant differences between practices are due to the habits of the doctors rather than those of the patients. In the long term, the doctor has a great measure of control over not only the quality but also the quantity of work that is done.

The various tables and figures (mostly derived from *Present State and Future Needs in General Practice*, 1983, RCGP) summarise the approximate distribution of conditions seen annually by a group of 4–5 GPs with 10 000 patients. As would be expected, about 65 percent of the consultations carried out are of short duration and are for self-limiting conditions (Fig. 1.2). Minor diseases (Fig. 1.3) do make up the bulk of our work, and this is the cause of much frustration to some family doctors who seem to resent the expenditure of their valuable medical time on self-limiting conditions. They do not accept that, although the illness appears minor to them, it may be a source of some anxiety to the patient. The reasons why patients present minor illness to a doctor are complex and may vary from the need for certification to irrational fears. The attitudes and skill of the GP in handling these consultations will largely determine the quality of the relationships with the patients in the practice. The better the relationship, the more fertile the soil for education to lead to less inappropriate consultations in the future.

While minor and neurotic illnesses make demands on the interpersonal skills of a doctor, acute and chronic major diseases (Table 1.2)

SETTING THE SCENE 9

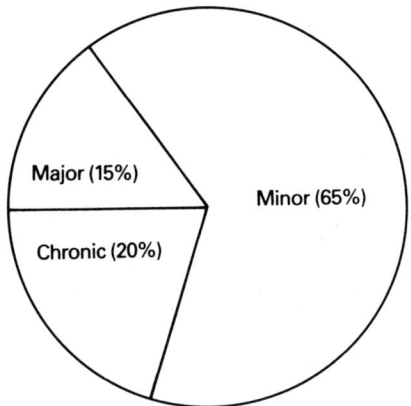

Fig. 1.2 Grades of severity of disease in general practice.

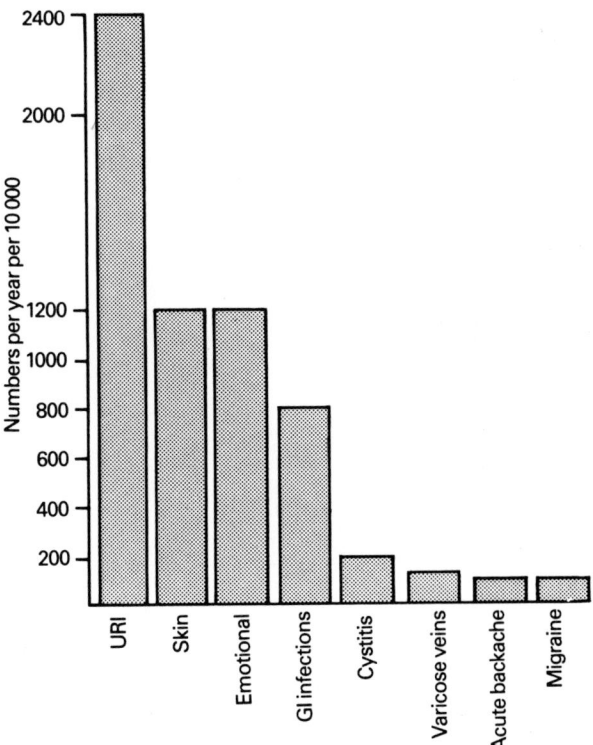

Fig. 1.3 Minor conditions seen in a year in a practice of 10 000

Table 1.2 Clinical events per 10 000

Acute (annual incidence)	Numbers per 10 000
Acute bronchitis and pneumonia	275
Acute myocardial infarction	35
Acute appendicitis	15
New strokes	20
New cancers	20
Severe depression	40
Chronic (annual prevalence)	
High blood pressure (plus 250 undiagnosed)	250
Diabetes (plus 50 undiagnosed)	50
Chronic psychiatric conditions	250
Chronic bronchitis	150
Asthma	100
Peptic ulcers	100
'Osteoarthritis'	250
Rheumatoid arthritis	50
Epilepsy	40
Thyroid disorders	25
Parkinsonism	15
Multiple sclerosis	10

Table 1.3 Social (pathologies) in a year in a typical practice

Condition	Numbers per 10 000
Elderly	
Over 65	1500
Over 75	500
Poverty (or supplementary benefits)	600
Severe physical handicap	280
Severe mental handicap	60
Single-parent families	at least 120
Divorce	20
Illegitimate births	12
Termination of pregnancy	20
Family planning	240
Juvenile delinquency	28
Adults in prison	16

require a considerable depth and breadth of medical expertise for their successful management. Good practice organisation is also needed in the long-term management of disease to ensure that patients are adequately monitored.

The incidence and type of social pathology (Table 1.3) in the practice will also influence the nature and amount of work done by the GP. The patient who is socially deprived is vulnerable to both physical and mental disease, and to manage the complete patient the GP must be knowledgeable and concerned about these problems.

Describing the content of practice in this way tells us only what is being presented to the GP. It tells us nothing whatsoever about how or how well GPs manage patients with these conditions, or even how we can judge how well they actually cope. Unfortunately there is little concrete evidence on which to judge the quality of care provided and hence the standard of practice of the provider. This lack of objective, proved yardsticks is likely to be longlasting and should not stop any of us from making our own considered judgements (as we do throughout this book!) about what constitutes good rather than bad practice and which of our colleagues we would consider as good rather than bad GPs. Rest assured, if we don't make such judgements ourselves others will soon come to make them for us.

THE DIVERSITY OF PRACTICE

Development and change have inevitably been patchy, and within the framework of the NHS there is now a tremendous variety of practices and practitioners. It is still quite common to find small practices run by one or two elderly doctors from inadequate premises and offering a minimal and unsatisfactory service to their patients. A few, however, are superb and their patients get highly personal and continuous care that is also medically efficient. These gems are normally to be found in rural areas, but not exclusively so. At the other end of the spectrum, large groups of eight or more doctors operating from health centres or purpose-built premises are becoming increasingly common. Organisational efficiency can benefit both patient and doctor, but inevitably medical care may become more impersonal and fragmented.

However, the diversity of practices is as nothing compared to the diversity of practitioners. Each doctor develops his or her own philosophy of care and then applies it in practice. Philosophies evolve from social and other subjective influences that are rarely tested objectively. Whatever makes doctors tick creates huge differences in procedures and leads to huge differences in costs and standards of care, quite apart from differences in possible iatrogenic consequences. Almost all measurable parameters show large variations among doctors, even within the same practices, e.g. referral rates to hospital consultants vary from 0.5 to 15 per 100 GP consultations — we can only imagine the range among doctors who would not even consider recording such figures.

Differences in the social and medical environments of practices obviously account for some of these differences, but they cannot explain variations on such a huge scale. As general practitioners have clinical autonomy and a considerable degree of control over their working conditions, it is their behaviour that must be largely responsible. The personalities and working habits of the doctors are the real determinants of the character and efficiency of any practice. The doctor's enthusiasm, drive, organisational ability, leadership and clinical skills are far more likely to influence the care a patient gets than any combination of environmental factors.

THE WAY FORWARD

In spite of the diverse types of practice that exist today, most of the problems, and thus the solutions, are basically the same. Whatever the practice setting or population characteristics, any improvement in the standard of service depends on the will and the ability of the GP to be objective about his or her work and to be disciplined and organised enough to initiate necessary change.

The aim of an efficient general practice should be to maximise the benefits and rewards to all the main parties involved. These are the patients, the doctors and the ancillary staff — though the government, which provides all the finance, must also be considered, as it has an interest in seeing that value for money is given. Unless all these parties are happy and satisfied, the practice will not be functioning optimally.

Patients expect effective and accessible care, delivered in as friendly and as personal a way as possible. Access to the service should be easy and appropriate, and the medical attention should be of a high standard and include preventative services and health education. Friendliness, concern and continuity of care are all features of good general practice, and the patient will be managed more realistically if the presenting complaint is assessed more fully in the light of the social and emotional environment.

General practitioners must be able to do a job that satisfies them intellectually in a setting that is comfortable and companionable. The workload must be reasonable and the financial rewards enough to attract doctors of high calibre to the discipline. Established practitioners must also feel financially secure, so that their clinical behaviour is not determined so much by their need to manipulate the system for their own financial gain as by rational appraisal of what might actually be best medically.

Practice organisation should allow the development of an effective general strategy for community care that carries the doctor beyond dealing, as best he or she can, with the immediate demands made by patients, into a simple and systematic search for their unmet needs and therefore to prevention as well as cure.

Ancillary staff such as receptionists, secretaries and practice nurses are so much an integral part of modern general practice that it is difficult to imagine any practice being able to operate successfully without their aid. Just like doctors, they will work better and more happily if they are well paid and are in a congenial environment where their special skills are properly appreciated and utilised. Adequate training and support are vital, as it is unfair to expect them to cope with the rigours of a demanding job without some special instruction. All too often GPs employ staff and then expect them to operate with the barest minimum of instruction and support, a situation that benefits none of the parties involved.

To satisfy all these requirements we need to abandon prejudices and preconceptions, so that the doctor can rationally change himself or herself. In the process, patient expectations, and the direction in which the practice is going will be remoulded. Doctor behaviour is the key to progress, and therefore deserves deeper consideration.

Doctor behaviour

Doctor behaviour is ordered by the concepts of professional conduct and status and the need to compete. These two motivating forces are often in conflict, and one can only assume that it was the need to compete that resulted in the almost universal and uncritical acceptance of the idea that there was a 'pill for every ill'. Or, as one old GP put it, "There's gold in them thar pills". To be fair, some of this behaviour was probably also due to professional ignorance about the efficacy of many treatments. In the days when there were very few active treatments available, it must have been very difficult to admit, even to oneself, that one was therapeutically impotent. Certainly, many a physician of yesteryear methodically bled patients to death while sincerely believing that he was actually doing some good.

Despite growing awareness within the profession of our therapeutic limitations, patients still tend to believe in the myth of the omnipotent doctor. This is the result of years of lack of education about how to cope with simple illnesses and the positive conditioning effected by doctors who prescribe rather than teach.

The reasons for the continuance of this doctor behaviour are complex. They include: inertia; a belief that a doctor is somehow less of a doctor if advice is offered rather than 'treatment'; difficulties with teaching or communicating which make prescribing the easier option; and a fear of losing patients and goodwill to high-prescribing competitors.

Our competitiveness and our views of professional status are also exhibited in our resistance to any encroachment by others on what we perceive as our field of work. Many GPs find it very difficult to believe that patients could possibly want to see or even benefit by seeing anyone other than themselves, so they are disinclined to delegate work to paramedical staff or to cooperate with other professionals such as social workers.

This independent streak has developed from the time when GPs really had only the placebo effect of their own personalities to offer and so were, as some still are, resistant to any objective evaluation of their work for fear that it might be found wanting. For a long time we have enjoyed popular prestige and have cultivated an aura of mystique, so that lay people regard us with awe and more uncritically accept our prognostications. The self-image of elite professionalism and individualism may have benefits in our dealings with patients, but it has become a dangerous delusion intraprofessionally, inhibiting ideas of audit either by ourselves or others. All too often the plea (defence is a better word) of clinical independence is used as an excuse for sloppy thinking and practice. Surely sensible, well-educated members of an elite group in society can talk to one another to agree on a common 'best-buy approach' to many of the problems, both clinical and organisational, that face us today?

To change our behaviour we must be able to reconsider our role, status and work, and plan rationally to place a greater emphasis on patient education and disease prevention. Delegation of work to and the involvement of paramedical and ancillary staff pose no threat to the doctor's status and can only enhance the quality of service given to the patient. Regular and frank communication between doctors, staff and even patients can help educate all concerned.

These developments do not mean that patient care has to become impersonal, remote or unfriendly. Part of the new ethos should be the friendly acceptance of the patient, even if the illness can be described medically as minor. We can deploy strategies to change patient behaviour, though this should not be done at the expense of the friendliness and trust that should exist between doctor and patient.

Standards of practice behaviour should be defined wherever possible. Every aspect of our work should be looked at, and there should be consensus decisions reached after full discussion between partners and any other staff who may be involved. Thus it is just as important for a practice to make decisions about the way patients are welcomed by receptionists as it is to define the practice protocols for the management of diabetics or asthmatics. Many GPs would be horrified at the thought that a practice should define and implement standards of care which were binding on its members. Standards imply some sort of audit to assess performance and this is seen as a threat. The usual cry is 'regimentation' and the expressed belief is that it is somewhat indecent to expect professionals to get together and actually agree to abide by consensus decisions on what might be best for their patients.

In the following chapters we will try to describe various strategies to improve practice efficiency and performance. We hope that you will find them as stimulating and interesting as we do, for we believe that general practitioners with their largely captive audiences, over whom they have effective medical control and ample opportunity to influence, can effect a revolution in health care. Competitive, treatment-orientated, dependence-encouraging work patterns can become more educative, disease-preventing and independence-promoting. Extra work generated will be balanced by work saved or delegated, and the sum total of the workload will become qualitatively very different. Less haphazard, better medical care will lead to better health in patients and greater job satisfaction and less stress for doctors and staff.

Section 2
Keeping the patients well and happy

Introduction

Keeping patients well (preventing or alleviating the effects of both disease and dis-ease) is what general practice is all about. Keeping patients happy is part and parcel of keeping them well. Without happiness or at least contentment with the medical service on offer, patient cooperation and compliance will be lacking. Patients cannot be kept well without being kept reasonably happy, though they can certainly be kept happy while being provided with a standard of care that will not keep them as well as possible.

The quality of the medical service offered to patients clearly has a profound effect on their health. Even the most cynical would have to admit that bad care can damage health, though some doctors seem reluctant to accept the corollary that good care can enhance health and wellbeing. We have no such reservations and believe that it is the family doctor who should carefully determine the most appropriate medical care, both for individual patients and the practice as a whole, and then deliver it in an acceptable and effective manner.

How acceptable the service offered appears to be to patients will depend on whether it satisfies their expectations. If there is a major divergence between the patient and the doctor about the nature of appropriate medical care, then the patient is very unlikely to be satisfied. To achieve a happy practice and at the same time provide a rational and appropriate service, doctors have to educate patients persuasively to change their ideas of what constitutes good medical care. This can be no mean task, as often patients will be very happy indeed with a service that is quite inappropriate to their real needs. GPs who would be, and are, judged by their peers to be appalling doctors can, nonetheless, engender tremendous affection and loyalty among the very patients whom, in a strictly medical sense, they are obviously failing. A doctor who does not 'believe' in immunisations and so refuses to immunise any of the children in his practice will persuade some parents that it is because he cares so much for their children that he does not wish to risk their suffering any side-effects. Others who prescribe reflexly will often be viewed as helpful and caring. As one new patient remonstrated after being offered advice rather than medicine for her son's snotty nose: 'But my old (real) doctor loved children. She never let any child leave her surgery without at least one bottle of medicine.'

Similarly, the cheery GP who copes with his own anxieties and lack of skill and knowledge by sending patients off for specialist opinions at the drop of a hat; by getting vast numbers of domiciliary visits done by consultants; by overloading Casualty; and by admitting far more patients than anyone else ever feels the need to, may well be regarded as a terrific doctor by his patients. He may be viewed as exceptionally caring and tremendously effective, a real decision-maker and a man of great influence in the local medical world (how else could he get so many specialists to work for him?). The fact that his patients suffer, among other things, more inconvenience, anxiety, investigations and iatrogenic disease and are getting inappropriate care is not recognised. Conversely, the conscientious doctor who is trying to do as much for his patients as possible and who keeps his referrals to a minimum may be regarded as an awkward customer if patients do not undersand his objectives.

More subtle than these obvious examples is the general belief among patients and doctors that the identification and treatment of physical disease is the GP's prime function. While this is an important function, uncritically acccepting it as the prime function results in much unnecessary investigation and treatment. This in turn generates inappropriate expectations in patients, who then aggravate the situation by their demands. To influence a belief such as this, it is vital that any changes in the organisation, style or emphasis of the services provided to patients must be accompanied by a great deal of education and explanation.

The way forward

Changing the direction of a practice in pursuit of the goal of better patient care while ensuring that all the needs of patients within the practice are accommodated and fulfilled is complicated and difficult. To achieve success, the general practitioner should aim to provide services with the following qualities:

1. Personal

The way the service is delivered and the quality of the emotional content of the doctor–patient interaction is usually more important to the patient than the quality of the organisational or clinical expertise.

2. Effective and efficient

This means good organisation and competent clinical care. There is no point in being terribly friendly and cultivating a good doctor–patient relationship if the patient then finds it difficult to get reasonable access to the system or is subject to indifferent or downright dangerous medical care.

From the purely medical point of view this may be regarded as the most important feature to get right, but it must be remembered that the best medical care may be thwarted by an uncompliant patient who is unhappy about the personality or behaviour of the doctor.

3. Appropriate

Every aspect of our work should be looked at critically so that its real value can be assessed. A high level of patient satisfaction with the service provided should not necessarily be accepted at face value. Patients are biased towards thinking highly of their doctors and, having got used to a practice's way of working, are not in a position to compare it objectively with another.

Ineffective and unnecessary treatment or investigation should be kept to a minimum, and patients should be protected from their own bad habits as well as the bad habits of other doctors. At the same time we must ensure that the best possible medical care is provided for those acute or chronic medical conditions which may benefit from treatment. Health education and disease prevention are activities that should take up a greater proportion of our time.

This list may be idealistic, but it does provide a feasible target at which to aim. Priorities in different practices will vary, and the social and geographical constraints under which the practice operates will also influence the character of the services provided.

Providing personal care

Although the term 'personal care' is much used, it can be difficult to determine exactly what is meant by it. We take it to mean a form of practice where patients have easy access to a doctor who has a considerable amount of background information about them and their families; who undertakes to provide the continuity of care essential for the formation of successful personal relationships; and who is able and willing to consider any problem that may be presented, whatever its nature. If the doctor is also welcoming, interested and skilful enough to allow the patient to express his or her problems fully, then the patient will be likely to regard the service as very personal indeed.

ONE DOCTOR OR ANY DOCTOR?

Many doctors and patients believe that personal care is best delivered by restricting the access of patients to one particular doctor. They argue that in this situation the largest numbers of close relationships will be formed and that better continuity of care and compliance will result. They also argue that access to other partners' opinions may fragment care and could harm the patients' confidence in their own doctor and his or her methods of working.

However, any advantages that may result from seeing only one doctor will as readily accrue to the patient, in a freely-consulting group, who exercises the right always to see the same doctor by choice. Such patients also gain the easily exercised privilege of consulting another doctor whenever they wish to. As nearly all patients have ended up on the list of a randomly selected, unknown quantity, who may or may not be capable of meeting their varied needs, this seems very reasonable.

Indeed, restricting patients to one doctor may be a policy designed to satisfy the needs of the doctor rather than of the patient. It prevents the doctor's ego being dented by a patient seeking a different or second opinion and it allows the doctor to practise in total isolation with no possible criticism from colleagues. They can only judge the public image the doctor is careful to present to them and not the reality behind it.

Being looked after by a practice

In large practices where patients may wander from doctor to doctor there are dangers that overall control of and responsibility for the patient may be lost and that conflicting advice might be given. It is reasonable to help patients to realise that there are advantages in seeing the same doctor most of the time, but this does not mean denying them the ability to see other partners for convenience or when there is a genuine need for another opinion. Accurate records and good communications between partners will help to fulfil the criteria of personal knowledge and continuity of care. Coherent practice policies on important clinical matters, particularly prescribing, will help the practice to present a common front to patients, so decreasing the risks of the doctors being 'played off' against one another or of the patient being given conflicting advice.

If communications and records are good enough, there is no reason why a patient should not be able to regard a team of doctors or even a whole primary health care team as 'personal'. A patient registered with a practice rather than a single doctor can then, by sampling the wares on offer, make an informed choice of doctor to provide the kind of day-to-day care they desire. Indeed, different doctors may well be known to patients as having differing abilities: 'Dr X is good at gynae, Dr Y is good with babies, but if your nerves are the problem see Dr Z.' — an extreme example, and ego-denting to Dr W.

In a group practice there will inevitably be variations in the way each doctor relates to patients. We all have some defects in our interpersonal skills but some doctors, and some patients, have more than their normal share of difficulties in relating to each other. Patients whose behaviour causes problems can be appropriately educated by the doctor, but it is not so easy for patients to educate a doctor whose behaviour is causing them problems. Therefore it is not unreasonable to expect doctors to educate each other if problems in relating to patients are identified. Of course, this type of interaction can only take place in an atmosphere of mutual trust and some degree of academic objectivity about performance.

If partners regularly discuss their problems, then situations where aberrant interactions have taken place are soon identified — usually with the doctor concerned drawing the partner's attention to the difficulty. A general exchange of views about how the situation arose and could have been avoided or better managed may then help to change behaviour. A little thought about the simplest of doctor–patient interactions can do a lot to reduce the number of incidents where patients get upset. A simple example is the technique for answering a telephone request for a visit to a patient with a minor illness. An immediate negative response may evoke a hostile reaction. However, if sympathy is expressed and a positive offer is made: 'I will certainly come if you really think it is necessary', one can then follow up with a suggestion that, as the symptoms are those of a simple cold or cough or whatever, then it is not likely to be serious and a visit from the doctor will not achieve much. The positive offer disarms aggression, enabling one to put a negative view.

Unless this sort of problem is talked about, little quirks of behaviour (and we all have them!) become ingrained habits and a cause of unnecessary friction with patients and partners, who then have to offer explanation and reassurance to more than the usual number of dissatisfied customers. A little thought and care given to altering doctor behaviour to increase patient satisfaction can produce a considerable improvement in the smooth running of the practice as a whole.

CARING FOR PATIENTS

Caring for and being interested in patients and their problems is a prerequisite of any successful doctor–patient relationship. If the doctor is seen as being remote or uninterested, then the degree of influence that can be exercised over the patient will be automatically depressed.

Our training is orientated towards the diagnosis and management of major disease, and the new entrant to general practice may, after a short time, find it very difficult to sustain interest in and sympathy for patients who present with minor illnesses. Sadly, some GPs never do manage to change their view of their role as doctors and deeply resent patients whom they percieve as wasting their valuable time with trivial matters. Such doctors may be very interested in and care deeply for patients with serious organic disease, but became completely switched off by the overanxious or introspective patient.

To be quite realistic, all but the most saintly GP will be irritated from time to time by patients who mindlessly or aggressively demand attention. Fortunately, such patients are in a tiny minority, though they do tend to loom large in our consciousness. Most patients have understandable and genuine reasons for their consultation, though a considerable degree of sensitivity and skill may be needed to understand fully the real reasons for some attendances.

Understanding why the patient has consulted

This presents one of the major intellectual challenges the GP has to face. Identifying and understanding the reasons for a consultation demands a considerable degree of sensitivity and a knowledge of the forces that determine behaviour in our patients. Having this understanding does not mean that we have to intervene in or try to solve every problem that is offered to us. It may well be more appropriate to teach the patient that a doctor's intervention is not needed and that they or some other agency should deal with the problem. A rational management decision cannot be made, however, without first gaining some insight into the reasons for the consultation. The presented cold may be inappropriate, but the intolerable stress that precipitated the consultation might be worthy of attention. Those who see this aspect of their work as boring either have not been able to identify the problems or are too cynical or insensitive to be bothered.

Sometimes, if there is difficulty in understanding why a patient has consulted, it is worth considering what has converted the idea of possibly seeing a doctor into the concrete act. As 80 percent of the population experience at least one painful and distressing symptom in any 14-day period, what leads most of them to self-medicate and only 1 in 5 to use the symptom as an excuse to consult? Zola identified a number of 'trigger factors' which can force an individual to seek medical aid:

1. The occurrence of personal crisis.
2. Perceived interference with social or personal relationships.
3. Sanctioning (a third party pushes — or is engineered into pushing — the patient to the doctor, so the blame for consulting is no longer the patient's).
4. Perceived interference with work.

For many patients it is the trigger factor and not the symptom which causes the consultation. The doctor must not confuse which social influences produced the symptoms and which triggered the consultation, or else the consultation is likely to be a failure. The doctor must also appreciate that the urgency of consulting may stem from the trigger factor and not the apparently trivial or long-standing symptom. Asking about the trigger will tell us more about why the headache or six weeks' standing must be seen immediately than asking about the headache itself will.

Cultivating tolerance and understanding

Doctors as a group have high levels of intelligence, motivation and education. Because of this we often find it difficult to appreciate how someone who is of limited intelligence, ill-informed and subject to adverse social circumstances will react in an apparently illogical manner to a relatively minor problem. We may have to make a conscious effort to imagine ourselves in the patient's position, trying to grapple with life's problems without the wherewithal necessary for their resolution. Mental exercises like this, if done deliberately and repeatedly, can increase sensitivity to the feelings of patients. The resulting understanding and awareness improves relationships and facilitates counselling and health education. The end result is hopefully not only a happier practice, but also a more effective and efficient one, with patients and doctors working to a common goal. We realise that no GP will have the skill or motivation to establish a full understanding of every patient's complaints. However, even a modest degree of succes is better than regular defeat.

Being tolerant and understanding does not mean that we have to be compliant to the point of acceding to all our patients' whims and fancies. It does mean that we try to understand their needs and respond appropriately. This may be by action or inaction, either of which might be contrary to the patients' wishes. The reasons for the action or inaction should therefore be carefully explained, so that even if patients are cross at the time, they will usually recognise the genuine interest of the doctor and later react accordingly.

The situation where doctors and patients regard each other as antagonists must be avoided at all costs. It is easy to feel a little paranoid and believe that patients are demanding or threatening. This may generate defensive and rejecting behaviour in the doctor, so no-one gains. The doctor will not be happy or satisfied with the job, and the patient will have to put up with indifferent and, often, inappropriate medical care.

Tolerance and understanding are so important to our work as GPs that we should be willing to audit ourselves and each other to make sure that we are behaving appropriately. Because we tend to work in isolation and rarely have a clear idea about each other's behaviour while consulting, it is all too easy to be complacent.

CONSULTING SKILFULLY

Patients seek help for almost any kind of physical, emotional or social problem. The time constraints of general practice make the routine, systematic history-taking of medical school and hospital quite inappropriate. The GP has to learn to be selective and flexible and to use a variety of consultation techniques to elicit information from patients and to cope with the wide range of presenting problems.

Information gathering

A straightforward physical complaint is easily dealt with by a selective question-and-answer technique. This is likely to be based on the old-fashioned SHIT system where the problem is delineated under S = symptom, H = history, I = investigation, T = treatment. The patient with emotional problems, however, may find it more difficult to talk to the doctor about feelings, anxieties and social strains. In some cases, patients may not have realised for themselves the true nature of their distress. Strategies therefore have to be developed to obtain the necessary medical information while allowing the patient both the opportunity and the time to express feelings and anxieties. An experienced and sensitive GP may be able to deduce quickly the nature of the problem and focus on it in a fairly direct way. On other occasions it will be better to allow the patient to set the pace and direction of the consultation. Time must be given to allow the patient to express ideas.

The use of broad opening questions, e.g. 'Is there something you would like to talk to me about?'; 'Where would you like to begin?'; 'What can I do for you today?', allows the patient to choose the subject to be explored. Similarly, the offering of observation, e.g. 'You appear to be very tense today'; 'You do look upset'; 'You have been crying'; 'You do look a bit angry; have I done something to upset you?', the use of encouraging words and sounds, e.g. 'Go on'; 'Tell me more'; 'Uh, uh'; 'Mmmm', and the appropriate use of silence can all help the patient to verbalise the real reason for attendance. All these strategies help to 'open up' the patient, in contrast to the more commonly used direct questions and closed statements which tend to shut down a consultation.

Although the finer nuances of the consultation are worthy of a book in themselves, the essence of good interviewing is to listen with evident interest to what the patient has to say, rather than to ask a series of routine, communication-inhibiting questions. A good consultation should reveal not only the nature of the illness, but also the patient's attitude to it. The patient's attitudes will determine whether the doctor's advice is likely to be accepted or rejected.

At the end of any consultation or sequence of consultations the patient should feel that the doctor has been told everything relevant. Patients cannot really be satisfied or happy if they are consistently unable to express themselves. It is incumbent upon the GP to develop the consultative skills to facilitate this process, allowing the efficient use of time to elicit economically all the relevant data.

Formulating a course of action

Once information-gathering has been completed, the consultation progresses to making a diagnosis and formulating a course of action. Although the lay mind does tend to jump directly from symptom to cure (with a natural prejudice for medicines), over the years patients have become increasingly unwilling to accept blindly a doctor's diagnosis and treatment. Nowadays most patients expect some sort of explanation and some relevant information. Misunderstandings and non-compliance are less likely to occur if the doctor has taken the trouble to explain his or her actions and to involve the patient in the decision-making. This also helps patients to feel that the doctor respects their opinions and accepts them as intelligent, responsible people. Condescension and offhand behaviour only breed resentment and, if things go wrong or if the patient feels that the service provided has not been appropriate, then the resentment may turn to aggression. The more a doctor involves patients in the decisions being taken about their care, then the more they will view him or her as being a competent carer.

Communicating with the patient

When trying to communicate information, ideas or feelings, the exact choice of words is very important, as it is all too easy for patients to misinterpret what we say. One example would be when an anxious parent presents a fretful child with a cold and the doctor says, 'Don't worry, there is nothing wrong.' What is meant is that the child is ill but that the illness is minor and does not require treatment. What is understood may be quite different, as the remark may be taken literally and the parent thinks the doctor is denying the presence of *any* illness. To the parent it is obvious that the child is ill, and the doctor's remark may be regarded as dismissive. The inexperienced parent will go away still anxious, possibly aggrieved, and certainly still ignorant of the nature of the problem. If the child is slow to get better, there may be aggressive requests for further consultations and treatment.

Had the doctor quickly and kindly agreed that the child was not very well, then given an explanation of the underlying infection and given reassurance that the child would get better without any treatment, the parent would have been likely to have been satisfied with the consultation.

This may seem a rather obvious example, but it is surprising how often dismissive remarks like this are made to patients. A little care and a little thought about how we express ourselves can make an enormous difference to the doctor–patient relationship.

Another barrier to communication that has to be overcome is that posed by various cultural taboos which discourage people from talking about topics such as sex, death and dying, suicide and mental illness. Doctors are subject to the same emotional constraints as patients, and often the doctor will collude with a patient to avoid discussing an embarrassing problem. Listening to tape recordings of consultations can reveal doctors deliberately shying away and changing the subject when the patient tries to open up and verbalise anxieties about a taboo area.

Patients can have a great need to talk about any facet of human behaviour or experience, whether or not the topic is likely to be embarrassing to the doctor. We must be brave and honest enough to analyse our own behaviour to ensure that we are not guilty of being evasive when faced with a problem that we find threatening. Very often we rationalise this evasion by convincing ourselves that it really was the patient who did not want to talk about it. Again we often need the help of fellow GPs to discuss these problems and to overcome them.

Most doctors feel that they are good at communicating with their patients yet studies show that about 50 percent of patients do not take their prescribed treatment or forget or reject their doctor's advice about changing their habit (See The Nuffield Provincial

Hospitals Trust, *Talking with Patients — A Teaching Approach*). Few of us, then, could fail to benefit from consciously trying to improve our ability to get information over to patients. To this end we should try to:

1. Provide better verbal information, avoiding medical jargon and pitched at the level appropriate to an individual's intelligence and circumstances.
2. Give out written, not just spoken, instructions and information that the patient, and family, may peruse and act on at leisure.
3. Check the patient's recollection and understanding of important points made, e.g. 'Now, tell me what you are going to do.'
4. For longer-term problems, careful supervision can help ensure compliance.
5. Self-audit by use of taping or, even better, video-taping of consultations which can then be critically appraised to improve communication skills.

When analysing and developing our consultative skills, it is important to keep a sense of proportion. What we do should be appropriate and, while we may encourage patients to reveal problems, we have no right to delve forcibly into their emotions. It is just as inappropriate to browbeat patients into telling us things they would prefer to keep to themselves as it is to stifle their self-expression by keeping firm control of the course of the consultation. Though it is important to learn different consultation techniques, sensitivity and an understanding of how patients are likely to feel and behave in certain situations is most likely to lead to successful communication. Empathy rules — OK.

Giving appropriate care

Caring in its widest sense is the basis of all general practice but, in our enthusiasm to be good doctors and to help our patients, it is very easy to dispense medical care too liberally, ineffectively or even dangerously. We should be willing to consider all the problems our patients bring to us, but we have to be selective about the way we respond. Being willing to listen to a patient's social and emotional difficulties does not mean that we have to take on the task of solving them. It may be far more useful to teach patients to be independent and to help themselves. Similarly, being willing to see patients with minor illnesses does not mean that we immediately have to reach for the prescription pad when it would be more appropriate to teach about self-care.

The ability to manage physical and psychological illnesses effectively should be amongst our most basic skills. After all, our training and experience should both lead to this objective. Yet, much of the treatment given to patients in practice, and anywhere else for that matter, is unscientific and irrational and designed mainly to satisfy the whims of our patients or ourselves. Part of the evidence for this is the vast amount of medicines such as antibiotics, linctuses, and diarrhoea mixtures, that are still prescribed for essentially self-limiting illnesses.

Patients need to understand our limitations and realise that self-care is a perfectly respectable activity. At the same time, they must be taught to seek help when this is appropriate (either for serious symptoms or screening procedures) and be able to appreciate that, when treatment really is necessary, then the best will be provided by a doctor who has maintained clinical skills and knowledge at the highest possible level.

A major source of patient satisfaction with the consultation is the relief engendered by the thoroughness of the doctor's consideration of the presenting problem. Thorough consideration mainly involves careful and thoughtful listening and selective examination — more often than not the 'laying on of hands' is performed for the patient's satisfaction rather than the doctor's need for further medical information. It does not necessarily involve any investigations or prescription.

INVESTIGATING SELECTIVELY

New entrants to general practice are inclined to over-investigate because of the insecurity engendered by hospital training, which directs them towards the exclusion of rare disease as a priority. They also feel a considerable need to arrive at a definite diagnosis — even if the diagnostic label is more a sop to their emotional needs than an accurate assessment of the patient — and feel inadequate if this is not achieved quickly. With maturity and experience comes the acceptance of the fact that it is impossible to make a clear diagnosis at every consultation.

It is worth repeating the truism that common diseases are common, so that a disproportionate amount of time and effort is not dissipated in a mindless search for exotic diseases. One of the strengths of general practice is the time-scale in which it operates. Patients are seen in a continuum and every problem does not have to be solved at one consultation. The passage of time can be used to help evaluate an illness, and a decision to investigate can be taken at a later date.

Thinking before testing

Before ordering any investigations, the following criteria should be considered:
1. Is this investigation necessary to:
   a. clinch an important diagnosis?
   b. monitor control of a chronic disorder?
   c. exclude a serious disease?
2. Will the results of this investigation determine the treatment or lead to a change in treatment?
3. Will the value of the results obtained justify:
   a. the inconvenience to the patient?
   b. the cost of the procedure?

4. Are there any special features of the investigation which require the patient to be provided with prior detailed instructions?
5. Can the specimen be delivered to the laboratory at a suitable time for them to process it?

Investigations carried out in self-limiting conditions, e.g. throat, eye, skin swabs; MSUs in women with recurrent cystitis, are usually of no value in guiding treatment, and the patient may well have recovered before any results become available. Routine pregnancy testing is another example of a wastefully irrelevant investigation. Despite an apparent, almost general, belief to the contrary, few doctors or patients can have any real difficulty in reaching a diagnosis of pregnancy purely on clinical grounds.

Other simple investigations should be on offer within the practice. Peak flow meters, for example, should be standard equipment in every doctor's surgery, and glucometers and ECG machines should only be absent as a result of a conscious policy decision and not as a result of inertia. ESRs and haemoglobins can also be easily performed by the practice nurse and help to improve the practice's standards of service and care. Similarly, if at all possible, patients should not have to travel to hospital solely to have simple tests performed. They can be saved both time and expense if the practice makes arrangements for the gathering and onward transmission of specimens.

Selective and judicious use of intrapractice facilities and of open access to hospital facilities enables the GP to investigate and manage many patients, thus increasing job satisfaction, reducing the load on hospital departments, saving the NHS money and saving patients both time and money.

Sporadic reviews of investigations being performed by the practice can be used to assess the clinical yield and cost – effectiveness. This might well lead to decreasing requests for some tests, though, where a particular test is shown to provide consistently useful information and to make the identification and management of an illness more efficient, its use might be increased.

PRESCRIBING SENSIBLY

Most patients seen by general practitioners do not need prescribed medication, either for the relief of symptoms or to treat disease. However, if a patient is anxious or distressed or seems to expect a prescription, if only to act as a talisman or touchstone, the doctor may feel the need to give one as a token of sympathy and willingness to help. With some patients, with whom communication is difficult, a prescription may be the only way the doctor can show some measure of understanding and a desire to please.

A doctor may give prescriptions for less exalted reasons. They can be used to avoid examining patients; to avoid listening to what the patient wants to say; to save time discussing a diagnosis; to save the time and effort involved in explaining any self-care measures the patient should consider instituting; and to keep the doctor in control of the consultation so it can be terminated at will.

Those patients who do need medication usually have to be left in sole charge of administering it. Its efficacy may depend on their appreciation of its importance, combined with intelligent and conscientious interpretation of the doctor's instructions. It is therefore very important for these instructions to be given clearly in the first place.

Depending on the condition being treated, it might be necessary to cover:

1. How the drug should be taken.
2. How it is likely to help the illness and how to judge whether it succeeds or not.
3. How long it should continue to be used and how the decision to stop it will be made.
4. What undesirable effects may occur and what should be done about them.
5. How important it is to take the drug and what is likely to happen if it is not taken.
6. If the drug is only to be taken 'as required', then what the indications are; how often the dose can be repeated; and the maximum total dose in 24 hours.

Acquiring good habits

In all human activities habits are often acquired without much conscious thought, and prescribing habits are no exception. Critical consideration of one's own prescribing habits can help to improve them, and may be aided by the following simple code of practice:

1. Prescribe nothing unless there is a clear expectation that it will materially alter the course of an illness or relieve suffering.
2. Use the cheapest satisfactory form of the drug that is available.
3. If the clinical indication is for a placebo, then make sure it is both cheap and safe.

4. Make sure the patient agrees to take the drug, understands what it is for and how it should be taken.

Good personal prescribing habits ensure maximum patient compliance with necessary treatment, with minimum patient risk from unnecessary treatment. They also help to educate people about drugs and encourage fewer patients to attend the surgery for problems they can then competently deal with themselves. By saving money, extra funds are made available for other NHS activities.

Of course, within a partnership it is as important for the practice as a whole to have good prescribing policies. Patients discuss their doctor's habits freely and soon know which doctor to consult to be certain of getting sleeping tablets, appetite suppressants, cough mixtures and what have you. Unless prescribing anarchy is to reign, consensus decisions have to be hammered out at practice meetings so practice policies on prescribing can be put into effect. Each doctor can then educate patients, secure in the knowledge that the other partners would support the action taken and would reinforce the advice should the patient seek to play one doctor off against another.

Many practices have policies not to prescribe barbiturates or appetite suppressants. From these it is a short and tremendously rewarding, though not necessarily easy, step to more general policies on, for example, non-prescribing for self-limiting conditions.

We would like to suggest that every practice sets itself the target of achieving prescribing costs which are half the present national average within the next five years. This is by no means an impossible task!

EDUCATING ABOUT MINOR ILLNESSES

An astonishing amount of time and money is spent in the treatment of minor illnesses. The fact that these are presented to the general practitioner at all indicates that a substantial proportion of the population are poorly educated about the nature and management of simple diseases. To be fair, you cannot blame people, particularly young parents, who have no knowledge of these matters, if they run for help when faced with an illness they have not experienced before.

The problem is exacerbated by the media and the profession itself who seem to spend a lot of time convincing the public that there is a cure for every ill. Though there is now quite a lot of literature which does try to educate the public about self-care, the most powerful educative force any person experiences is the action taken by their doctor. If treatment is routinely prescribed, then the patient rightly learns that the consultation was necessary and that the disease needed medical treatment. Advice without a prescription can have the opposite effect.

Influencing future behaviour

To illustrate this, let us look at how three different doctors might handle the same consultation.

The patient Mrs Winge (aged 30 years) has just moved from Hainault. She brings her spoilt only child, Wayne Winge (aged five years) because he has yet another cold and cough. (You can make up your own mind about who is the real patient.) Wayne is snotty, sniffs a lot and has offensive sleeves to his jacket. However, he looks well and promptly sets about demolishing the surgery. Mrs Winge witters on about Wayne's colds, his tonsils, his eating habits and his nocturnal cough which keeps her awake.

1. Dr Blunderbuss Aged 50, this doctor runs a five-minute appointment system. He always finishes on time in spite of seeing one or two extras, and knows how to keep patients in their place. Through long experience he has found that his patients appreciate a prescription, preferably with many items on it, and are impressed by the apparent ease with which hospital consultations are arranged for them. He quickly takes command of the consultation, asking a few direct questions and supplying some of the answers himself. After a brief examination he prescribes penicillin, promethazine (Phenergan) nocte and paracetamol (Calpol). He assures Mrs Winge this will make Wayne better. Time for consultation: four minutes.

2. Dr Thunderthighs This mature part-time general practitioner has recently returned to practice after taking a few years off to raise her own family. She used to be a clinic doctor and is a bit unsure of herself. She listens sympathetically to Mrs Winge who makes hay while the sun shines and carries on at some length. After some difficulty in catching Wayne, a careful examination is performed. She finds that Wayne appears to be deaf to a ticking watch and has a red throat. A throat swab is taken, and after consulting MIMS she prescribes some Septrin. As some of Mrs Winge's anxiety is transferred to her she asks to see Wayne again in three days' time and also refers him to the ENT specialist for audiometry. Time taken: twelve minutes.

3. Dr Smart-Alec A doctor aged 35 who 'sort of' believes in

Balint. He is critical about the patterns of work in the practice and consequently irritates his partners on occasion. He is human, though, and has been known to prescribe penicillin for a sore throat late on a Friday night. He listens to Mrs Winge but takes control of the consultation as time runs on. He tries to find out if this consultation is really for some other problem, or what her anxieties are about Wayne. When a quick examination reveals a simple cold, he explains to Mrs Winge that Wayne is basically very healthy and that like many other children of his age he will suffer frequent colds but will get better as he grows older. No treatment is offered. Time taken: six minutes.

Effect on patient behaviour These three consultations will all affect the future behaviour of Mrs Winge (Fig. 2.1).

Consultation 1

Anxiety about Wayne
↓
Consultation
↓
Treatment
↓
Mrs Winge satisfied but not educated. Prescription confirms belief that colds need medical attention.
↓
Next incident

Consultation 2

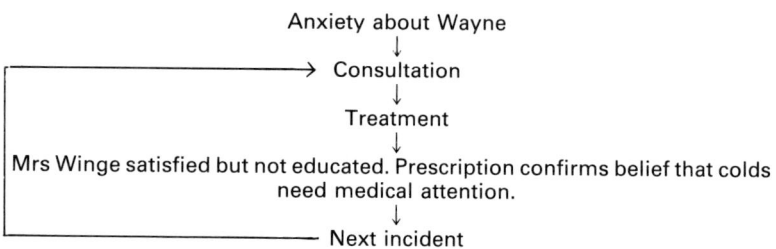

Consultation 3

Anxiety
↓
Consultation
↓
Explanation but no treatment. Mrs Winge is reassured and, while she may be unhappy that no prescription has been given, she learns that colds do not need medical attention.
↓
Next incident: considers self-management

Fig. 2.1

The same strategies are valid for the management of visits (Fig. 2.2). Imagine the scene.

Sunday, bloody Sunday It is 1 p.m. and lunch is about to be served. Mrs Worryguts phones about little Karly who is aged three years. She has been off colour for a day and now she is 'burning up'. The presence of a runny nose and a cough indicate the probable diagnosis, but Karly's mother is insistent that a visit is necessary.

A. Dr Sourpuss His wife moans about how patients can smell lunch in the oven, so he mollifies her by saying he will be back in 20 minutes — just time for the potatoes to cook — and dashes out. On arrival, in rather grumpy mood, he fires off a few terse questions and does a very brief examination. Karly just has a cold and sore throat, he says, as he hands over two sachets of amoxycillin (Amoxil), writes a prescription and leaves in a huff before Mum can ask any questions. He is home in 18 minutes, and is a likely candidate for a coronary.

B. Dr Smoothie He takes the call, gives advice and then enjoys his lunch. He visits later in the afternoon, at his convenience, to find that fluids and aspirin have settled the child, who is now playing. He examines the child and teaches her parents about normal illnesses. No prescription is given.

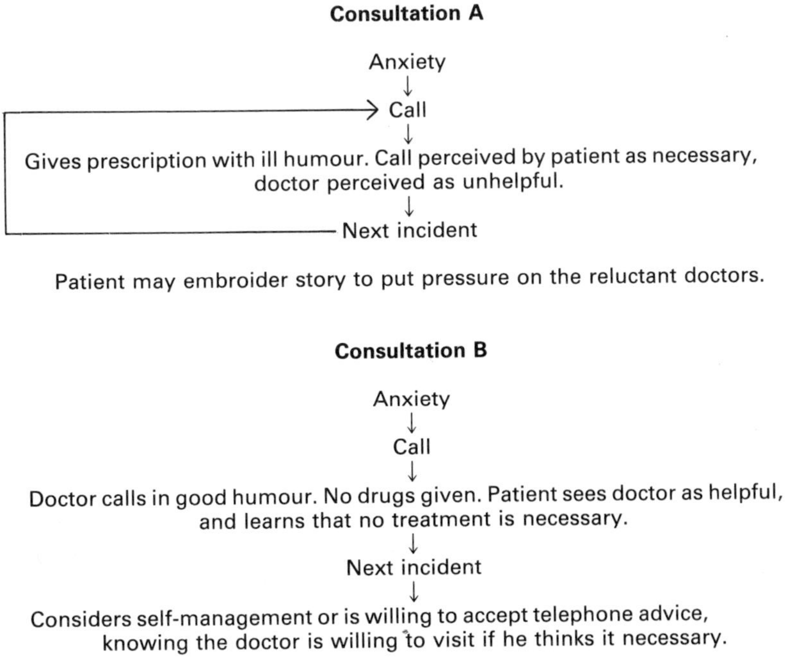

Consultation A

Anxiety
↓
→ Call
↓
Gives prescription with ill humour. Call perceived by patient as necessary, doctor perceived as unhelpful.
↓
Next incident

Patient may embroider story to put pressure on the reluctant doctors.

Consultation B

Anxiety
↓
Call
↓
Doctor calls in good humour. No drugs given. Patient sees doctor as helpful, and learns that no treatment is necessary.
↓
Next incident
↓
Considers self-management or is willing to accept telephone advice, knowing the doctor is willing to visit if he thinks it necessary.

Fig. 2.2

If a patient's expectations are not going to be fulfilled, then an adequate amount of explanation is needed. A bald statement that 'Penicillin is not necessary' will not suffice if their previous venerable and kindly GP always gave penicillin. Instead of changing expectations, you are more likely to produce the belief that you are an idiot or that you must be gaining financially in some way by not prescribing. A few simple facts about the nature of virus infections and the dangers of using antibiotics too freely are usually appreciated and the patient may well conclude by saying, 'Why didn't anyone tell me about that before?' This is time well spent, though sometimes the exercise will have to be repeated once or twice before the message gets through. In a few cases the message makes no impact at all though, if the doctor remains consistent, a surprising number of patients will eventually appreciate what is happening. For these patients low anxiety levels will still result in fairly frequent attendances; the difference is that attendance is for examination and verbal reassurance and not for prescription. Although the doctor's time is not saved, the NHS's money is.

The object of teaching is not just to keep patients with minor problems away. It is to help patients to consult appropriately. It is equally important to make it clear when advice should be sought, e.g. for a child with a persistent fever for no obvious reason, the child who is vomiting a lot; and to be seen to be willing to see people when they are worried.

Let us look in more detail at two common minor illnesses:

Upper respiratory tract infections

These viral infections rarely need antibiotics for their resolution. Even tonsillitis and otitis media can get better without the magic pink medicine. This is hardly surprising, as they are mostly caused by viruses too. Even when tonsillitis is streptococcal in origin — and which of us can differentiate between a streptococcus and a virus on clinical grounds? — penicillin will only shorten the illness by a day or so.

Likewise, there is plenty evidence that a substantial number of cases of otitis media do not need treatment, though in practice one does need to use one's judgement. It is perfectly justifiable to prescribe an antibiotic for a child with an acutely bulging drum and a fever, or to a patient with filthy tonsils and painful cervical nodes, even though the worst-looking throats are likely to be glandular fever. What is not justifiable is reflexly to prescribe penicillin for sore throats and amoxycillin for sore ears. Not only is there no clinical need, but the practice will condition patients to come for a bottle every time they or a member of their family gets the same symptom again. A short consultation plus prescription will have to be repeated time and again over a lifetime, whereas a longer consultation (though not much longer) with explanation and no prescription will lead to far fewer repeat performances.

There is also no justification for the millions of prescriptions for medicines like aspirin, paracetamol, cough linctuses and antihistamines doled out annually to try to alleviate some of the symptoms of respiratory infections. All of these preparations can be obtained over the counter without a prescription. They are all freely available household remedies, and our terms of service do not require us to prescribe such simple nostrums. If patients want to take them, then they can buy them by going direct to the chemist and bypassing the doctor. Putting these medicines on prescription invests them with a mystique quite out of proportion to their likely therapeutic value.

Advising patients with colds to take plenty of hot drinks, aspirin/paracetamol or whatever similar preparation they have in the house, and to use Vick, will satisfactorily conclude most consultations. Patients who say they have tried a wide variety of medicines for their cold already and would like something stronger can be sympathised with as you point out that they are providing support for your view that nothing will make much difference. Common sense will determine which patients on low incomes might benefit from the placebo effects of a cough syrup, or what have you, on prescription, though sympathy in itself should not be an excuse for ineffective prescribing. Barrack-room lawyers who demand their 'rights' to a prescription can either be told that no such right exists or be given a simple prescription that would be cheaper to buy than to pay a prescription charge for.

Perhaps it is wise not to teach patients to use even these simple remedies unthinkingly. All too often patients are told to take aspirin every four hours for a fever. It is not explained that this does nothing to hasten a cure and is only helping the symptoms. Most patients, and some doctors, believe they are fulfilling some important therapeutic function by suppressing any fever. In fact, as a normal body response to infection, fever has a biological function and acts to slow the rate of viral replication. It is reasonable to try and relieve the aching and vile headache of a high fever and important to hold down the fever of a child with a history of febrile fits, but for everyone else the simple statement 'Take aspirin every four hours for the fever' should be changed to 'Take aspirin every four hours if needed for the pain and aching.' This does not take long, and it is surprising how many patients cheerfully abandon all medication when they realise that it is not really hastening a cure.

Diarrhoea and vomiting

In spite of all the evidence that has accumulated in the literature that drugs of any sort have little or no part to play in the management of gastrointestinal infections, many GPs blithely prescribe on. As a result of this prescriptive conditioning the public has been led to believe that medicines are necessary to relieve the unpleasant symptoms. They are not.

As with URTIs, education and explanation should be clearly given so that not only can the presenting attack be managed correctly, but also so that subsequent attacks, in the extended family or among friends, can be properly dealt with, often without further medical advice. The patient or family must understand that:

1. Whatever the causal organism, most attacks settle quickly on their own within 2–3 days.
2. Limiting intake to clear fluids only will decrease vomiting.
3. Antidiarrhoeal mixtures, such as kaolin and pectin, have no proven place in therapy though, apart from distracting attention from the more essential management of dehydration, they are harmless and, if desired, can be bought from the chemist. Stronger drugs may actually be harmful as they can interfere with the body's own mechanisms for clearing out the 'bugs' and so can prolong the attack.
4. Antibiotics are not necessary.
5. Fluid replacement is all-important, and the doctor's instructions for rehydration must be followed carefully, particularly in the case of infants.
6. If vomiting or severe diarrhoea persists or if fluid intake is insufficient, then the parents must make sure that the child is seen again by the doctor.

With children the advice given is doubly important. Apart from the educational value, correct management can actually be life-saving or save an unnecessary admission. It is not enough to say 'give lots of fluids'. Details of suitable fluids, frequency with which they should be given and the target input to be achieved must be made clear. Prescription without clear advice is dangerous. Prescription with clear advice is better. Simply explained, clearly understood advice without any distracting prescription is best of all.

From these two examples it can be seen that appropriate care of minor illnesses is 90 percent reassurance, advice and education. Reflex reaching for the prescription pad is costly, inappropriate, counter-productive and possibly dangerous.

The same principles apply to all minor illnesses, and each doctor should have a repertoire of considered statements to present to the patient. Being creatures of habit we repeat the same stock phrases over and again; how much better if they are truthful statements that will let both patient and doctor get the most out of the five or six minutes they have together.

The result of the consultation will then be fed back into the lay system and the practice community's store of knowledge. There, if social ties are strong, the information will be used to deal with other patients without recourse to any medical opinion.

MANAGING CHRONIC ILLNESSES

The long-term management of chronic illness and handicap is properly the job of the general practitioner. Specialists, social workers, nurses and other professionals may be involved, but the responsibility for the patient must lie with the GP. This responsibility is not a nominal one, and care should be active and continuing, otherwise it becomes fragmented.

Most, if not all, hospital out-patient departments are cluttered up with chronic patients who return time and again to be seen by a succession of junior hospital doctors ignorant of their cases. This certainly does not constitute continuity of care. These pointless visits take place either because no-one is willing to take the responsibility of discharging the patient or because the consultant is so disillusioned that he or she fears that if the patient is discharged no proper care will be available from the GP. Regular care from a good GP would certainly be more convenient for the patient and would be likely to be more emotionally satisfying and medically effective as well.

If patients are found going back and forth to hospital for no good reason, a tactful letter may be sent to the consultant concerned, asking if attendance is still necessary. Most would then be delighted to pass the patient back to the GP. Sometimes regular specialist checks are needed, though then a system of shared care can operate, with the GP doing most of the checks and providing continuity between the occasional hospital visits.

Though a considerable amount of organisation is needed to provide good long-term care for the chronically sick, this need not involve much in the way of extra workload. The usual excuse of being too busy to undertake extra work does not hold water, because it is extra thought that is needed rather than more time.

Once we decide to make a positive effort to improve long-term care then careful planning should make care effective without being too onerous. The main principles of good care are:

1. **Arranging regular reviews at realistic intervals**

Patients who are chronically ill tend to fall into two categories: those who come too often and those who attend erratically, usually only when something has gone wrong. The over-enthusiastic — often doctor-encouraged — attenders clutter up surgeries. The frequent visits may actually be counter-productive because the patient is being seen so often that the doctor may not undertake a proper review of the clinical situation when this is necessary. The transaction is likely to become quick and stereotyped, fulfilling social needs rather than medical ones.

Every practice has its supply of regulars who come once a month or so to have a chat or pick up some tablets. Once the habit is established it is difficult to break, as the doctor may feel guilty about then rejecting the patient. Some courage is needed to alter the status quo by gradually lengthening the time between appointments. This has to be done with tact, so that the patient does not feel rejected.

The opposite problem is the patient who attends a few times, then disappears for a long time, only to be rediscovered by chance or when something has gone awry. Many of these patients are fatalists who feel well and so do not believe anything can be wrong with them. Many others, however, do not reattend because the doctor has not explained why their regular attendance is important, what it is trying to achieve and what beneficial effect it is likely to have on them.

2. **Identifying patients for recall**

Ideally, a complete diagnostic register would allow the identification of patients with any chronic disease. The notes could be checked by receptionists or clerks at prearranged intervals to see which patients had not attended for review. Those patients could then be sent a reminder. Realistically, this kind of register is beyond the capabilities of all but the most obsessional of doctors.

However, it is quite easy to keep a record (card index or loose-leaf) of a limited list of conditions. All partners have to agree which conditions merit regular surveillance and then, as they identify cases, enter the names in the register. Once the register has been compiled, the record envelopes of all patients with a recorded condition can be easily retrieved for checking. Such checks should not be too frequent, or else they will become a major administrative chore.

In the not too distant future many practices will be using microcomputers for this purpose (see p. 231).

3. Using a precise repeat prescribing system

Another method of checking patients with chronic conditions is by using the repeat prescribing system (see p. 227). It will not help pick up diabetics on diet alone, but most other chronically ill patients are on drugs. Monitoring accurately allows patients who have not been seen for a reasonable length of time to be asked to reappear — on pain of having their little white pills cut off.

Repeat prescriptions should only be issued for a fixed time or a fixed number of repeats. When either criterion is exceeded, then the patient is asked to come and see the doctor. Our system operates in this manner, but to be successful it needs a certain amount of self-discipline on the part of the doctor. It is all too easy to scribble out a prescription when one is a bit rushed or not looking forward to seeing a particular patient.

4. Having clear ideas about the medical objectives

Having gone to the trouble of organising regular reviews, it is important to have a clear idea about the purpose and form of the checks. Each disease ought to be evaluated and a management protocol defined. For a single-handed GP this requires thought, but for a group practice the protocol should be thought about, discussed and then agreed by the partners (see p. 237).

This does not infringe clinical freedom or destroy the supposedly vital individualism, so beloved of all doctors. What it does allow is each member of the practice the freedom to influence his or her partners so that a reasonable and reasoned consensus view is arrived at. It allows the partnership to have its own standards so that patient care is determined more by current concepts of good medicine than by the vagaries of fate which determine the standards, or lack of them, of the individual doctor the patient is exposed to.

When partners do get together to argue out a protocol, a great amount of detail is not needed. What is important is to establish a consensus on such matters as base-line investigations; diagnostic and treatment criteria; what follow-up checks and at what intervals.

So far we have concentrated on the purely medical aspects of chronic care because it is so easy to be very friendly with the patient, and have a good relationship, while allowing medical disasters to develop in front of one's nose. Having said that, the importance of social and emotional support for the chronically sick should not be underestimated. This does not mean that 'more of the doctor' is necessarily the right prescription, though the dependence that this can produce is often pleasurably ego-boosting. It does mean that the doctor must take the trouble to talk to the patient and any caring relatives about the nature of the illness and the prognosis. A realistic, though better optimistic than pessimistic, view of the future can help maintain the effort of being independent and cooperation in achieving medical objectives.

Any social or emotional problems need to be explored and appropriate help sought. A good working relationship with the nurses and local housing/social services can be a great help in resolving many of these difficulties.

REFERRING JUDICIOUSLY

Annually, 11 percent of the population are inpatients; 15 percent are new referrals to outpatients; and 20 percent self-refer to Casualty. These figures are awesome and undoubtedly represent some of the work that could and should be carried out in general practice.

While there are many valid reasons for referral to hospital for admission, opinion or investigation, the ease and convenience of the referring doctor or the rejection or punishment of the patient should not be among them. Good care can take time, and we should be willing to see patients often enough to maintain a satisfactory level of supervision. The dying and many chronic patients can be looked after quite adequately at home if the GP and the rest of the primary care team are willing to do their best. Selected coronaries, strokes and other acute major conditions can also be lookd after at home if the GP is prepared to revisit and reassess. Even performing minor ops in the surgery can decrease the hospital workload and give the patient a better, quicker and more convenient service, while not greatly increasing the practice work. Unnecessary referrals and admissions are unfair to the patient and costly for the NHS.

Taking pride in not making unnecessary referrals should not hinder referring when this would be to the patient's advantage. An objective and unselfish evaluation is needed in every case. In cases where the GP has not thought of getting a second opinion, a patient's request for one may come as quite a surprise. The doctor may feel upset, hurt, bewildered, rejected or even angry. The doctor's feelings notwithstanding, the patient's wishes should be calmly explored.

Writing good letters

On average a GP will write eight referral letters a week, and the best ones will be brief and to the point explaining what the problem is, what investigations or treatment has been carried out, why referral is taking place and what is expected from the consultant. The letter should make it clear what the reason for referral is (second opinion re diagnosis; help with new or modified management techniques; reassurance of the patient; giving the GP a respite from a demanding patient; to effect some procedure the GP cannot effect) and under what conditions the GP wishes to take back the patient's future management.

It might be thought that professional pride would be incentive enough to keep standards of referral high, though there is another equally important reason. Hospital doctors judge a GP's quality mainly by the quality of referral. Such judgements may be superficial, but they greatly influence the way hospital doctors react to individual GP's requests and the ease and appropriateness of access that the GP's patients will be granted. Although it can only be an opinion, we believe a good GP's patients are likely to get a higher standard of hospital care whenever they need it.

To assess the appropriateness of one's referrals is not too difficult. The practice secretary can produce copies of the referral letters and the notes of the previous 50 or more referrals. The doctor should then find the answers to the following questions:

1. Are my reasons for referral legitimate (see above)?
2. Could I have better managed any of these patients myself?

3. If receiving them, would I have found my referral letters helpful?
4. Is there any evidence that I use referral to reject patients or that my choice of consultant is deliberately punitive?
5. Do I have any dependency needs that are being fulfilled by some referrals?
6. Do I have any specific illness phobias resulting in inappropriate referral?

Once the outcomes of the referrals are known, then a further analysis will be fruitful, particularly in providing some idea of how appropriate and useful to the patient the referral actually turned out to be.

Emergency admission criteria and outcomes can be usefully audited in much the same way. Comparisons among partners of numbers of patients referred or admitted in any 3 months–1 year period can also be very instructive.

Preventing disease

With a captive list of patients, 90 percent of whom will be seen in any five-year period, the GP is in a unique position to carry out health education and screening programmes. If inclined to do so, practitioners can use their power and influence to motivate patients towards healthier lifestyles and to protect them from the detrimental effects of a number of diseases.

Unfortunately, many doctors feel unable to cope with the demands already being made on them for disease treatment. They are therefore not willing to go looking for extra work. This is sad, because not too much extra work is actually involved and what there is should be highly productive in terms of cost-effectiveness and patient satisfaction.

Health education is delivered in the context of the six-minute consultation and depends on using available time more efficiently. Screening and the delivery of preventative programmes, e.g. antenatal care, immunisation, are really organisational problems. After the planning stage the practice team should be doing the bulk of the work, and again the GP should be little affected. Indeed, if antenatal care were subject to critical scrutiny (see p. 238), most practices could safely see patients less often yet do better by them.

EDUCATING ABOUT HEALTH

Public health education is not as successful as it should be. The bulk of the population seem to be easily stampeded by media-inspired panics yet far more difficult to influence by more subtle, medically accurate, positive campaigns.

There seem to be two broad schools of thought among patients.

One group feel that they are responsible for their own health and see disease as a result of lifestyle. The other group are fatalistic and tend to blame external factors for their illnesses. This second group will only consult when they are ill and will often refuse to change their own behaviour. In general, social classes 1, 2 and 3 are more likely to feel responsible for their own health and to use preventative facilities, while social classes 4 and 5 are more likely to be fatalists. As many preventable illnesses are more prevalent in social classes 4 and 5, it is unfortunate that they are less likely to respond to health education and to use prophylactic services.

At one extreme we have the muesli and kaftan set, into yoga, Zen Buddhism, vitamins and goodness knows what else, while at the other we have the flat cap brigade whose Uncle Fred smoked 100 a day until he was run over by a bus at the ripe old age of 96. Thankfully, most patients are in between these extremes and can be influenced by their GP in a way they would never be influenced by general measures.

Educating patients about disease prevention requires patience, tact and obsessiveness. In the surgery the patient is normally open to suggestion, and firm advice coupled with information may be acted on. Advice without information may be regarded as didactic and rejected, so the interaction should be at an adult-to-adult level and not at a parent-to-child level. The patient should be involved in any decision-making, as this enhances the feeling of personal responsibility so necessary for any action.

As only a certain amount of information can be absorbed at any one time, chat sessions should be kept short and the facts presented as clearly and concisely as possible. Most patients cannot retain more than two or three items of information after talking to their doctor, so a handout (see p. 233) can be very useful in reinforcing and expanding what has been said.

To aid information retention and to prevent the patient feeling threatened, if many aspects of his or her lifestyle need modification simultaneously, only one subject should be tackled at a time. Success can lead to further modifications; failure can help avoid counterproductive nagging. It is important for the doctor to keep a sense of proportion and to know when to leave well alone. It is quite pointless trying to change the behaviour of the obese matron whose notes reveal a long saga of fruitless diets and inappropriate prescriptions for anorectic drugs. Similarly it is kind to ignore the fag the 70-year-old bronchitic has put in the ashtray, even as he berates you for doing so little to help his breathlessness. In addition, goals must realistically reflect the community in which the doctor works; what is appropriate to the stockbrokers in Weybridge is likely to be inappropriate amongst the out-of-work buffer girls from the steelworks in Sheffield.

Taking every opportunity to impart information

Being alert to the opportunities for health education in every consultation helps patients to believe that the doctor really is interested in their welfare and can help to change their behaviour. Smoking, drinking and exercise habits can be asked about, almost routinely. Current contraceptive use should be recorded for all women between 15 and 50, and this same group should be made aware of the importance of being rubella positive; having five-yearly smear tests, and of undertaking regular breast self-examination. Young parents should be given information and encouragement so that their children achieve as good an uptake of immunisations as possible, and so on. The possibilities are endless, and information-giving should become a deeply ingrained habit.

This educative process should not just involve doctors but should permeate the activities of the entire practice. Every member of the primary care team should be willing and able to give advice and information appropriate to their status. Communication and teaching within the practice should be good enough to ensure that there is agreement about what patients are to be told. Besides talking to patients, receptionists, for example, can help by giving out leaflets on topics such as cervical cytology or breast examination. They can also put up posters or notices in the waiting room — as long as these are simple and only tackle one subject at a time, they can be quite effective.

However, authoritarian posters are best avoided, as they tend to be negative and may invoke hostile feelings in the captive reader. Far better that they should be pleasant and cajoling — 'Thank you for not smoking', 'If you have been waiting longer than half an hour please see the receptionist', 'Are you due for a cervical smear?'

Some sophisticated practices have even installed small projectors which automatically display a succession of slides to the captive audience in the waiting room. How much this will influence patients is not known, but it does allow practices to make up programmes suited to their particular population needs.

SCREENING CONSCIOUSLY

The concept of screening patients for risk factors or presymptomatic disease is becoming ever more popular with the public and politicians to whom it is transparently obvious that the earlier any disease is found and treated the better. Some doctors also hold this simple belief either sincerely or because they have a vested interest in maintaining a livelihood based on screening. Unfortunately, though preventing disease certainly should be better than treating established disease, experience has shown that screening programmes only sometimes produce the expected beneficial results.

Before embarking on any screening project within a practice, a critical assessment must be made of the aims, expected benefits and cost in time and money. The basic criteria for any screening procedure (see Table 2.1) should be considered, though the most crucial questions to be answered are:

1. Does detecting the disease or condition in its early stages really alter the prognosis?
2. If so, is the alteration sufficient to justify the screening effort and the early treatment costs?

Outcome (what happens to the problem when it has been picked up) not process (the number of cases the screening programme is picking up) is the important factor. Too many arguments for screening hinge on the justification on the process, not the outcome. The case for paediatric surveillance, for example, is particularly weak on this point.

Table 2.1 Basic criteria for a screening procedure

1. A suitable disease or diseases
    a. reasonably common
    b. with serious effects
    c. with a fairly long presymptomatic phase
2. A suitable test or tests
    a. simple — rapidly applied, preferably by paramedics
    b. acceptable
    c. giving reproducible results — little observer variation
    d. sensitive — few false negatives
    e. specific — few false positives
    f. economy — applicable to large numbers of patients and should be cheap
3. Suitable treatment
    (Effective treatment must be available and, furthermore, there must be an advantage in treating the disease at a stage before the patient would otherwise seek advice.)
    a. offering a better chance of cure
    b. in the earlier stage needing less severe treatment than if the disease had progressed
    c. relieving a disability for which the patient would not otherwise have sought help

Despite these reservations, there are areas where practice screening programmes are totally justified medically, are cost-effective and well worth instituting. At present the case is very strong for:

1. Determining rubella status in all nulliparous women and immunising those who are seronegative.
2. Providing an intrapractice service that ensures all women aged 20–60 have five-yearly smear tests.
3. Recording blood pressures in all patients aged 35–65, every five years.
4. Providing effective antenatal care to all pregnant women so that any complications are picked up as early as possible.

Though they are not screening, the other preventative measures well worth vigorously pursuing are those of achieving an immunisation rate as near 100 percent as possible and of offering a high-quality contraceptive service.

There is really no case for instituting a comprehensive screening programme for adults and only a poor case, despite the bandwagon merrily rolling along at present, for developmental surveillance. Though sophisticated screening techniques may be having some impact on survival rates from cancer of the breast, annual examination of the over-35s by a doctor has not been evaluated. Even if it were shown to reduce cancer death rates, the evidence would have to be of overwhelming benefit to justify the massive medical effort that would be needed — monthly self-examination (after being taught by a trained nurse or reading a Health Education Council booklet) would be more likely to be the answer.

The case against developmental surveillance

As it is currently assumed to be a 'good thing to do', yet we believe it is not, let us look at the developmental surveillance arguments in a little more detail (Table 2.2).

Before the lack of evidence in favour of developmental surveillance became clearer, two of our partners were specially trained in this form of screening, and all small children in the practice were routinely screened. After several years we evaluated our results and felt that the useful yield was so low that the time and effort was not worth our while. We shall not offer this service again until the following areas of doubt have been clarified:

1. Comparison with a control group with children randomly allo-

Table 2.2 Developmental surveillance

For	Against
Parents feel they are getting better and more personal care. Improves doctor–patient relationship. May reduce number of 'acute consultations'.	False positive results may cause a lot of anxiety and worry. False negative results may inappropriately reassure parents and doctor so that abnormalities are then not dealt with until later than they would have been if no screening had taken place.
Health education advice is more easily given and accepted.	The greatest need and least interest is among those who will not attend. They can be given advice by the health visitor or when they come for routine consultations.
High immunisation rates are achieved.	Can be as easily achieved without a surveillance programme.
Abnormalities are picked up and dealt with so every child has the opportunity to achieve its optimum potential.	The majority of the conditions picked up are minor. No evidence that these would not be picked up anyway or that they can in any case be effectively or better treated.
Doctor enjoys the regular contact with children and feels fulfilled.	Does this justify the time and effort needed? Is the screening programme within the competence of a well-trained health visitor?

cated into surveillance and non-surveillance groups.
2. Assessment of the value of the programme by result of outcome and not of process. Outcome to be shown to be beneficial to the child and the parents and a definite result of the programme.
3. Normality defined and the sensitivity and specificity of the screening tests evaluated.
4. The diagnosis of the suspected disorders tested for repeatability.
5. Evidence that health visitors are not as good as doctors at picking up speech, vision and hearing problems which seem to constitute the bulk of discovered conditions.
6. Evidence that side-effects are not greater than the benefits.
7. Evidence that costs and work input will provide a reasonable return.

Our remarks are directed at a complete doctor-based screening service and do not mean that all screening efforts are pointless. All babies should be examined soon after birth by a doctor. This will be the GP's responsibility if the baby is delivered in a GP unit. Even if the baby is delivered in a consultant unit, baby examinations are usually carried out by the most junior doctor of the medical team and it may be reasonable for the GP to look at the baby at any postnatal visit.

A practice might also like to establish a system for checking infants for treatable conditions that are still missed with great regularity e.g. dislocated hips and undescended testes. In our practice we have recently picked up no fewer than three boys over five years of age with undescended testes, yet they had all been screened by clinic medical officers. Virtually all children are seen by their GPs, so one could use the system of putting stickers on the cards when a particular examination has been done. The absence of a sticker alerts one to the fact that the patient has not been screened.

We do appreciate that many practices feel that the social and emotional as well as medical rewards of surveillance make it worth pursuing. We have presented a rather one-sided argument, not to try and win it by default, but to try to illustrate how we make policy decisions and so all move in the same direction.

Screening practices should coordinate their efforts with those of the District Health Authority (DHA) clinical medical officers and health visitors. Non-screening practices should maintain a high level of clinical awareness when seeing children for whatever reason; ensure that whoever is screening their children on the DHA's behalf refers or reports back any abnormalities found; and ensure that all parents know to bring their child if there is any worry about deafness, squint or any other developmental problem. Education by the doctor, midwife and health visitor during pregnancy, in the postnatal period and when a parent attends with the baby for any intercurrent illness will all help to achieve the aim.

Organising effectively

Providing a realistic preventative programme within the practice is most rewarding. Standards of patient care are enhanced, patient satisfaction with the service the practice provides is increased and there is greater job satisfaction for doctors and staff. A streamlined organisation, making the maximum use of the talents of directly employed and attached primary care team members, ensures that the time and effort involved is low enough not to prejudice the rest of the service. Also, if maximum advantage is taken of the opportunities that exist to earn fees for item-of-service payments, any costs of the enhanced service that have to be borne by the practice will be at least partly offset.

While a single-handed or small two-partner practice might find it most cost-effective for the doctors to do all the work, most other practices will find that appropriate delegation is the key to success.

Identifying patients

As 70 percent of patients consult at least once a year (women in the reproductive age group consult on average five times each a year), a doctor methodical and disciplined enough to consider prevention for a few seconds before every consultation can tackle patients as and when they come to the surgery for other matters.

Good records (see p. 207) can act as a reminder for screening and other procedures. The front of the record envelope (and/or the summary card and contraceptive record card) can be marked by colour-coded stickers which show, for example, when the last smear or BP were taken and when, by implication, the next ones are due (Fig. 2.3). The back of the record envelope can be reserved solely to record immunisations (Fig. 2.4) and so can also be easily scanned before any consultation to check if a jab is due. Inside the envelope a distinctive contraceptive record card can be used to record rubella status, contraceptive usage and the date the next FP1001 becomes due. Faithful recording allows any patient who has not been appropriately screened or advised to be easily identified.

This method is cheap and does not involve intense bursts of activity. Once the practice gets into the prevention habit, 90 percent of the population can be screened over a five-year period, then as easily rescreened over the next five years. Patients who do not go along for a smear or vaccination when advised to can be tactfully asked why whenever they next consult — their misgivings can be allayed and further explanation can be given if needed. Patients who would not normally respond to invitations to come for preventative procedures, and in whom there is likely to be the greatest incidence of positive findings, can have smears or BPs taken without any real effort on their part.

For more comprehensive screening programmes, an accurate age–sex register is necessary (see p. 220). It allows the identification of groups of patients who are at risk or who merit screening. They can then be approached directly by the GP. Microcomputers can provide an accurate and easy to use age–sex register, but are no more capable

FEMALE SURNAME			FORENAMES	Smear 81 NAD 1982	
Date of Birth	Single / Married / Widow		National Health Service Number		
Address			Doctor's Name	Committee's Cipher & Stamp	
Tel. No.					
Subsequent Addresses					
Tel. No.					
Tel. No.					
Tel. No.					
Occupations	Year		Occupations (Note changes and insert year of change)	Year	FORENAMES / SURNAME
Date of Death 19					
Cause of Death					
Doctor's Signature					

Fig. 2.3 Front of a record envelope. We use a red sticker for BP and a green sticker for cytology screening. The stickers are available at no cost from Winthrop.

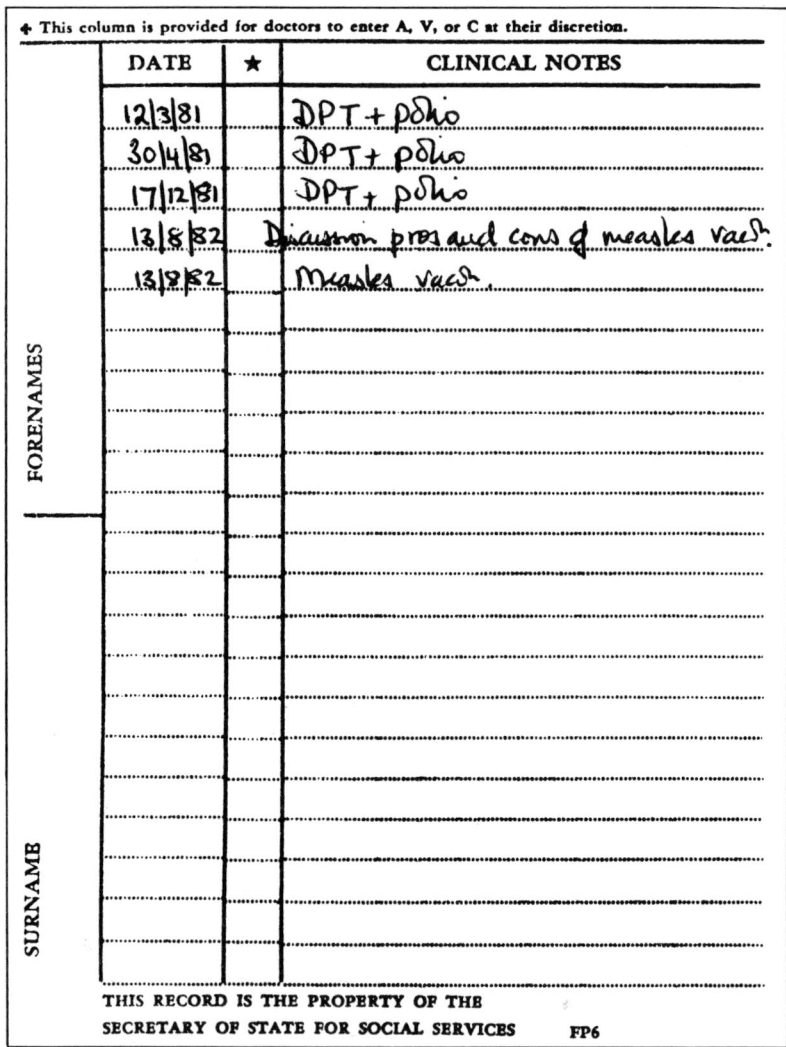

Fig. 2.4   Back of a record envelope. Reserving this for immunisations allows parents to be gently reminded if any vaccinations have been missed.

than the manual register of actually getting patients to accept their invitation and attend.

Delivering the goods

How then can a cost-effective, smooth running preventative service best be provided? There are four main areas worthy of consideration:

1. Contraceptive care With a systematic approach, contraceptive advice can be offered appropriately to all women in the reproductive age group. A service can be taken to the poorly motivated who are often most in need of it.

However, actively seeking out patients is of little value unless the practice has a comprehensive and up-to-date service to offer them. One reason for this is that effective long-term use of contraception depends to a large degree on patient confidence and satisfaction with the standard of care received. Whatever doctors may think about method safety, many patients do have fears and reservations and these can be allayed by the knowledge that their doctor is looking after them carefully. From the doctor's viewpoint this might well mean carrying out procedures such as smears, breast examinations, and rubella titres which, while not strictly connected with contraception, do appear to the public to represent a high standard of practice and do indicate to patients that the doctor is interested in their general wellbeing rather than in just handing out contraceptives.

Good intrapractice care should comprise:

a. An up-to-date, well-informed doctor able to fit both diaphragms and coils. Viewed by the patients as an informed authority yet flexible enough to allow patients to choose their own methods (without too much manipulation).
b. A special contraceptive record card in the notes (see p. 213)
c. An integrated screening programme so that rubella status is checked in nullips; five-yearly smears are performed on all patients; and all patients are offered a leaflet or advice on self-examination of the breasts.
d. (Possibly) an intrapractice family planning clinic run by a doctor or by a family planning trained practice nurse who can carry out Pill, coil and diaphragm checks as well as fit diaphragms and take smears.

The income generated by FP1001 and FP1002 fees will more than compensate for any time and effort expended. Seeing a woman twice a year to check her blood pressure and give her a prescription for the Pill pays more than looking after her for everything else for the entire year. Even fitting just one coil a week within the practice will provide a superior financial return to any kind of weekly DHA or hospital sesssion.

2. Antenatal care While the GP can have no direct means of increasing the number of pregnant patients within the practice, the provision of antenatal and postnatal care lends itself to efficient, timesaving organisation that also can lead to greater patient satisfaction.

Points to consider to maximise the benefits include:

a. All pregnant patients should be booked as early as possible. Reception or secretarial staff should be responsible for all the paperwork and raising all the necessary forms/cooperation cards/ blood tests and so on.
b. Keeping a central record of the date patients book and their EDD. About 1–2 months after the EDD has passed, secretarial staff check if the patient has attended for postnatal examination and, if not, send the patient a reminder.
c. An antenatal clinic should be established in the practice as the most efficient way of concentrating the care and time of doctors, staff and patients.

   Ancillary staff can check all weights, urines and even BPs before the patient is seen by the doctor or community midwife — who could be invited to attend to help provide a practice service extending throughout the whole pregnancy.

   The health visitor could also help follow up non-attenders and run relaxation classes, mothercare classes and so on. Either the health visitor, midwife or practice nurse could carry out a long interview/advice session with each first-time attender.
d. The partners should decide their clinical policy on antenatal care (see p. 238) so that if patients see different doctors or team members they will not get conflicting or confusing advice. A special record card should be kept in the notes and used meticulously to record information such as haemoglobins, rhesus antibody checks.

   Every effort should be made to provide personal antenatal care so that patients have time to talk about their worries and problems and not get processed rather mechanically. A wider-ranging service might be better appreciated than the ritual proddings we seem to indulge in at present.
e. At every postnatal examination contraception should be discussed and consideration given to the taking of a cervical smear. After the examination a member of staff fills in the FP24 carefully, and FP1001, 1002 and 74 if appropriate. All such forms shoud be sent to the FPC at the end of each month.

3. *Immunisation*   Whether for children or overseas travellers, this

is one preventative activity that every practice must pursue with vigour. The clinical benefits are enormous and there is a reasonable, direct financial return for the effort. With a little organisation it is easy to achieve vaccination rates of over 90 percent. Any practice which does not know whether at least 90 percent of its under-2s are being vaccinated is, quite bluntly, failing to provide reasonable care.

Virtually all the work can be delegated to suitably trained staff who are, in any case, much better than doctors at carrying out routine procedures carefully. Of course if the practice nurse, for example, is carrying out all the vaccinations, then the doctor remains responsible for her actions and must ensure that she is fully trained and competent. Regular teaching sessions will be necessary to achieve this.

Teaching of and discussion with the HVs is also important, as their active cooperation is vital for any practice scheme to succeed. One partner should act as a vaccination authority to organise care and training, to deal with any problems that may arise and to monitor the practice's performance. Other points to consider to maximise the benefits include:

a. Encourage every member of the team to take every opportunity to educate parents about the importance of immunisation.
b. Run a well baby or vaccination clinic in the surgery with the health visitor and practice nurse in attendance. Getting vaccinations done while at the well baby clinic is more convenient for parents and will result in higher attendances than can be achieved by anonymous local authority clinics.
c. Allow the practice nurse to vaccinate during most, if not all, of her working hours. Again this can be very convenient for parents and stops them 'forgetting' to come back.
d. Devise a system to identify and follow up all children who have missed a vaccination (see p. 223), so that the only children not vaccinated are those whose parents have consciously decided that they shall not be vaccinated.
e. Devise a system to ensure all prospective travellers get comprehensive advice before they go abroad (see p. 225).

4. *Screening* Different procedures will make different organisational demands. In general, unless a practice is particularly well organised, doctor identification and immediate motivation of patients will be a better prospect than any age–sex register based campaign.

a. **Rubella:** All young nullips whose notes show no record of rubella vaccination should be asked if they were vaccinated for this at school. If they are certain they have, then their card can be annotated accordingly. If they are uncertain then, regardless of any clinical diagnosis of rubella that may have been made in the past, they should be persuaded to have a rubella titre carried out (Fig. 2.5).

Doctor identifies patient and writes out form.
↓
Patient goes to nurse to have blood taken then phones receptionist in one week for result.

Rubella positive	Rubella negative
Patient informed and notes annotated.	Patient again attends nurse who vaccinates after advising no pregnancy or risk of pregnancy for 3 months post-vaccination. Fills in form to claim for payment and records vaccination on back of record envelope.

N.B. If the woman is at all reluctant to have a bloood test, then we will offer vaccination there and then. This will do no harm even if she is already rubella positive.

Fig. 2.5 Screening for rubella

A keen practice, cooperating with the schools' medical service, might use their age–sex register to send every girl a birthday card on her 10th birthday. This card would contain an invitation to attend for rubella vaccination and the nurse could easily monitor and send reminders to non-attenders.

b. **Smears:** All women should have five-yearly smears, from the onset of sexual activity to the age of 60. For a 2300 patient list this would mean doing 126 smears a year or 2–3 a week for one doctor. For every 400 smears done in this way one case of cancer of the cervix could be prevented.

Although doctors can obviously take some smears themselves, the procedure does take a few minutes and could be easily neglected in a busy surgery. An intrapractice smear clinic run by a suitably trained nurse is very useful. Any patient identified as due for a smear is advised to book for it at reception as she leaves. This takes seconds and is likely to result in a high smear uptake.

When smear results come in, the record envelope and summary card are suitably amended. Patients are told their smear should be repeated in five years and discouraged from having unnecessary smears in the meantime.

If a practice wished to screen comprehensively for carcinoma *in situ*, then the smear clinic nurse could also be responsible for the organisational aspects of the screening programme. Patients would be identified from the age–sex register and sent personal letters inviting them to attend the clinic. Reminders would be dispatched to non-attenders, and in some cases the nurse might even do home visits to take smears.

c. **Blood pressures:** All patients between 35 and 65 should have their BP taken at least five-yearly. Without doubt this is best achieved by all partners regularly taking BPs on all 35–65-year-olds whose notes do not show they have had one taken within the previous five years.

To make the system more effective, the doctor needs some sort of reminder to check BPs during routine consultations. The easiest way to do this is to have a sticker of a distinctive colour on the notes with the date of the last BP recording on it. The absence of the sticker should induce a Pavlovian reflex in the doctor to take the BP.

It is interesting to note that, when one studies trainee consultations on video, whenever the going gets tough the trainees automatically take the BP. Unfortunately this does not seem to be always recorded in the notes and it is strange that it is the 'in and out' consultation where a BP could fruitfully be recorded which is the very time when it is not done.

Non-training practices may feel that this is one area in which they can easily make a start towards practising preventative medicine.

Being accessible

Practice organisation is a major determinant of the level of accessibility. Different doctors and different patients have particular views about what constitutes good access. A single-handed doctor with a small list and no appointment system may consider that his or her patients have total access, forgetting that the surgery is only open for 2–3 hours a day and contact with a doctor for the rest of the day may be difficult to achieve. Another practice may have a tight appointment system, but doctors may be present on the premises most of the day — offering accessibility of a different type and quality.

As the number of doctors within a partnership or premises increases, so then does the average distance patients have to travel to the surgery. Access to a car becomes very important, and the elderly and lower social classes are put at a disadvantage. These groups are also handicapped by having less easy access to telephones and so experience greater inconvenience in making appointments. Furthermore, they are less able to cope with complex organisations and may not have the intelligence, language or forcefulness necessary to negotiate with or persuasively appeal to receptionists to get urgent appointments or home visits.

For the elderly, natural sympathy and understanding does help smooth the path to the doctor. For some, particularly young male adult members of social classes 4 and 5, a tendency to become aggressive under stress causes most receptionists' natural reserves of sympathy to evaporate quickly. Though, to be honest, in the short term, aggression too will speed the journey to the doctor.

Monopoly practices and large groups do not need to provide late-evening surgeries to hold patients. Lack of access to a GP in the evening may create difficulties for people who work all day, though this can be more than compensated for in large group practices where doctors are available all day and so can be seen at any convenient time.

Open access to practice nurses who can then get an instant medical opinion for problems they cannot deal with also allows for free access to medical care for the patient, yet more appropriate access to the doctor. Some audit of the work of the practice nurse is necessary, however. Inappropriate use of the nurse — as a means of bypassing the system — may occur. More worrying is that the nurse may be offering inappropriate or inaccurate advice on topics of which she knows little. Training must be given to avoid this.

MAKING APPOINTMENTS

Though appointment systems (see p. 191) are fashionable, they are not necessarily appropriate for every practice. When the number of patients using a surgery is so small that demand at any one time is never great, then an appointment system may be a discardable luxury or even a positive disadvantage. Where the workload is heavier or the waiting-room space is limited, an appointment system becomes necessary to avoid overcrowding and chaos in the surgery. Flexibility is the key to success with either system. The small surgery may still find it convenient to have a few appointments for special purposes, like medical examinations or coil fittings. The surgery with an appointment system must also be able to cope with patients who have not got appointments, yet who feel their problems are urgent.

An efficient and flexible appointment system works to the advantage of doctors, patients and receptionists (see Table 2.3). An inadequate and inflexible system may well still be of great benefit to the doctors while aggravating patients and stressing receptionists.

Any system is doomed to failure if the demand for appointments consistently outstrips the supply. Receptionists are then put in the invidious position of trying to keep the patients happy while protecting the doctors from their demands. The receptionists then come to be seen by the patients as the regulators of demand (the dragon at the gate) and may come under attack. Feeling somehow that it is their job (perhaps even having been told by the doctor that it is their job) to make the demand fit the supply, the receptionists may not communicate their difficulties to the GP who, safely shielded in a consulting room, can conveniently ignore any hassle going on in the

Table 2.3 Appointment systems

	Advantages	Disadvantages
For patients	Convenient appointment times. Reduced waiting times. Less queueing and less crowding in waiting room. Surgeries run throughout the day.	May act as a barrier. Need access to telephone or may have to get to surgery 2 times to be seen once. Elderly and lower social class patients may not be able to cope with system.
For doctors	Workload evenly spread. Able to make and keep other commitments which require reliable timekeeping. Surgery facilities fully utilised. Allows forward and flexible planning.	More staff needed. May feel guilty because not instantly available to patients ('I'm God's syndrome). Extra calls may swamp telephone system. May cause conflict with receptionists.
For staff	Workload evenly spread. Doctor on premises for most of the working day. More challenging and stimulating job.	May cause friction with patients and doctors if demand outstrips supply.

office.

Every appointment system should be kept under regular review and the pressure assessed realistically. A fair and achievable aim would be to maintain a supply of appointments allowing patients to see any doctor within 24 hours and their own doctor within 24–72 hours. One responsible doctor or senior receptionist should look at the appointment books routinely and assess the state of forward booking. If appointments are getting booked up too far in advance, then surgeries have to be extended or extra surgeries slotted in to cope. Regular extension of surgery time implies too high a workload or too little doctor time to deal with it. More surgery time or a new partner should be considered, while gradual changes in work patterns can be effected. In our opinion a doctor rather than a receptionist should be in charge of making the supply of appointments fit the demand.

Coping with urgent cases

While most patients can easily book their appointment at least a day or two ahead, there will always be a certain number who think that their complaint is urgent and that they need to be seen the same day, if not sooner. To accommodate them, some appointments should be left unbooked until the current session, or receptionists should be allowed to slot in urgent non-appointments at the end of surgeries. Spaces may be left free in each surgery, or in larger practices a designated day duty doctor can run a morning and evening surgery, the appointments for which are kept free until that day. Whatever the system, there will still be difficulties in reconciling some patients' concepts of urgency and the consulting slots available — on the whole the patient should be allowed to make the decision and, if the doctor disagrees, suitable education should be forthcoming.

One disadvantage of making access very quick and easy is that patients may develop false expectations and not bother to try and book up in advance. Being accustomed to getting in to see the doctor quickly and at their convenience, they may get quite upset if they are thwarted in any way. The successful management of this will largely depend on the skill of the receptionists. It is not unreasonable to respond to the first request for an appointment by making an offer of a time for the next day or later, even if there are appointments free on the current day. This should help to communicate the idea that it is reasonable to think at least 24–48 hours in advance. If the patient baulks at this, an offer can be made for the same day, though it should be made clear that he or she is being fitted in as an urgent case. Labelling the record with some sort of flag lets the doctor know that this particular patient has been fitted in as an urgent case, so that this can be discussed if in fact the appointment has been made inappropriately.

Receptionists must also be on the lookout for the patient who is too compliant. An example is the man with chest pain who meekly accepts an appointment for tomorrow without communicating his problem to the receptionist. This can usually be avoided if the receptionist concludes the transaction with a question like 'Is that alright?' or 'Are you quite sure that is suitable?' which allows the patient an opportunity to verbalise any difficulties.

This can be represented as a flow chart (Fig. 2.6).

HOME VISITS

Home visits, so much a feature of British general practice, are now decreasing. Twenty years ago a GP might easily have done ten to twenty visits a day, yet nowadays the average is probably five or fewer. The big reductions have occurred in chronic visiting and in visiting for minor ailments, such as upper respiratory tract infections. Resistance from doctors, appointment systems and the in-

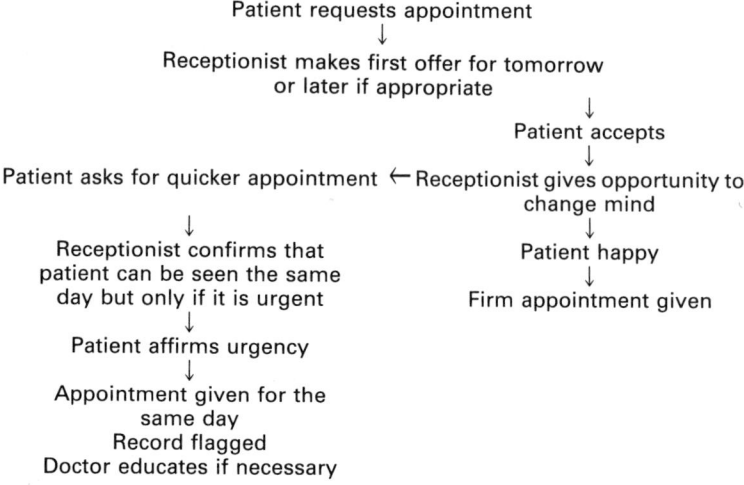

Fig. 2.6 Making appointments

creased availability of cars have all produced a shift towards consulting in the surgery.

Though time-consuming, home visits do have a definite role in the work of the GP. It can be useful to see inside our patients' houses from time to time because this can reveal a lot about the family and social conditions. On the other hand, however, it is not particularly useful or economic to go there time and time again. All sorts of factors have to be taken into account when deciding if a visit is justified: how ill the patient is, the availability of transport, the weather, the emotional state of the caller, family problems and the patient's expectations are all relevant.

Once again receptionists may get caught between patients asking for visits and doctors who grumble. Their job is made easier and patients made happier if requests for visits are accepted without too much of a fight and any necessary education done later. If there is serious doubt about the necessity for a visit, the matter should be referred to a doctor. Receptionists should never be put in the invidious position of having to refuse a request for a visit. Patients may accept that sort of decision from a doctor, but they become very resentful if it is made by a non-medical person.

Many visits for children with rashes or respiratory tract infections can be avoided if the parents are offered a quick consultation in the surgery. First, they should be reassured by the receptionist that bringing the child out will not be harmful in any way. Then they should be told that they will not have to hang around the surgery with their feverish, fretful child but will either be put straight in to a doctor or parked in a spare room until the doctor is available (this counters any arguments about not wanting to bring the child to the surgery in case diseases are passed on to waiting patients).

These cases do not take up much time and can usually be fitted in as a 'quickie' between normal appointments. If this is all done quickly and efficiently, parents soon learn that this is better for them as well as saving the doctor the trouble of making a visit.

COVERING OUT OF HOURS

The adequacy of out-of-hours cover is an even more emotive issue for patients than the supply of appointments or the doctor's willingness to do home visits. Again, accessibility is the crucial factor, and it must be easy for anyone to contact their doctor (or deputy) in an emergency.

While telephone-answering machines and large rotas are a great boon to doctors, their usefulness should not be at the expense of patient access. Calm people in daytime can find it difficult to cope with answering machines, so every doctor on call should be certain that anxious, frightened and confused patients can reach them, without undue delay or added distress, at any time of day or night. Complicated messages or 'round robins' of answering machines are not legitimate ways of limiting workload.

This, however, is not the same as saying that the doctor is obliged to respond to every demand as the caller wishes. Patients must be able to get appropriate medical advice and visits without a struggle, though it is up to the doctor to decide whether to visit or not. When deciding when a visit is justified, medical criteria are not the only ones to be considered. Anxiety, low intelligence, inadequate health education in the past and social problems may all be factors in precipitating a call for help and may only be allayed by the doctor's presence. Kindly, considerate interest in the caller's problems helps to generate confidence and trust, even if some visits are then done on emotional rather than medical grounds. Once patients realise that the doctor will visit when necessary they are more likely to allow future decisions on telephone advice or visiting to be made by the doctor (see p. 39).

Another factor to consider when providing out-of-hours cover is the degree of familiarity likely to exist between the patient and covering doctor. Some argue that the ideal situation is for the patient's own doctor always to be available (continuous rather than continuing care), though this situation, with its overwhelming disadvantages for the doctor (e.g. boredom, tiredness, overfamiliarity with problem patients), is as likely to impair as enhance patient care. Indeed, few patients would really expect or wish their own doctor to be continually available and are happy to accept alternative advice in an emergency.

Whether this same degree of tolerance extends beyond partnerships or small rotas, whose members soon become easily identified, is more debatable. Certainly, deputising services are now commonplace (over 40 percent of GPs use them) and, provided their response times are reasonable, seem to be quite acceptable to patients. Indeed, some patients prefer them to their own GP, as they are virtually guaranteed a visit if they want one and they can easily be used for a second opinion. Their disadvantages are: lack of continuity of care; lack of access to the patient's medical records; lack of patient education by deputising doctors; and provision of, often, totally inappropriate care by hospital-orientated deputising doctors. These are not really recognised by patients and all too often unrecognised or conveniently ignored by GPs using deputising services.

To be honest, we do not believe that lack of continuity of care or access to records matter much but the provision of inappropriate, prescriptive and dramatic care most certainly does.

Unlike deputising, large GP rotas do provide cover by experienced GPs. In theory this should lead to better care than deputising can provide, but in practice if often does not. This is mainly because patient access to the covering GP may be poor, and visits, other than for obvious medical emergencies, difficult to gain from doctors with no interest in keeping other GPs' patients happy. Also, there are rarely any controls over the standards of medicine being practised by the rota and one or two bad GPs can undo much of a practice's efforts at good care and patient education. With mutually enforced standards, a large rota could give good out-of-hours cover — as such standards are difficult to develop and adhere to even within well-motivated partnerships, it seems to us highly unlikely that any rotas are likely to develop them.

Ideally, then, GPs should do their out-of-hours duties within their own partnerships or in small rotas. If the pressures of work make it difficult for the patient to get a reasonable, good-humoured out-of-hours service, then deputising may be better for all concerned.

Promoting comfort and convenience

Patients are extraordinarily tolerant and often put up with discomfort and inconvenience without complaining. This is no reason for taking advantage of them.

In the past, general practice was under-funded and the poor general standard of buildings and furnishings was understandable, if not quite acceptable. This situation has now changed, and rent and rate reimbursements make it eminently practical financially to erect purpose-built and well-furnished accommodation. Any practice that works from dingy or cramped premises should actively consider alterations and additions to improve them.

The quality of surgery accommodation does affect the quality of service given to patients. It is difficult to have an efficient office, run special clinics or even ensure a reasonable degree of privacy if the size of the surgery is hopelessly inadequate. Any practice that aspires to giving its patients the very best possible service must therefore look critically at its premises to see if they are up to the job.

SITING THE SURGERY

The problems associated with building a new surgery are beyond the scope of this book. Due consideration must be given, however, as to how patients are going to get to the surgery. An ideal site would be close to the densest areas of housing and on at least one bus route. If the practice is scattered over a wide area, then a choice might have to be made between limiting the practice area or setting up branch surgeries. On the whole, these are administratively difficult to manage and militate against a cohesive service. If at all possible, it is better for a practice to have only one surgery.

In rural areas where communications are difficult, it may help if surgeries and other clinics are timed to fit in with public transport schedules. Some practices have experimented with the idea of providing a minibus service to bring patients, particularly the elderly, in from outlying areas. This can be expensive, but might just pay for itself if it saves the doctor a lot of visits or having to set up a branch surgery.

Motorists too have to be considered, and adequate parking space is needed. This is often a problem in urban areas and can be the cause of some difficulty and ill feeling. If there is a major problem, the local authority might reserve some parking for patients in a nearby road or car park. If nothing else, they should be pressured into catering for disabled drivers.

Within the surgery, planning should take account of the needs of the disabled (particularly making everywhere accessible by wheelchair) and of young mothers with prams. It is better to have a fairly secure pram parking area than the chaos caused by prams in the waiting room — especially on clinic days.

KEEPING UP APPEARANCES

First impressions of a practice are gained in the reception and waiting areas, so these should be as clean and comfortable as possible. Reception is more personal if there is no glass or other barrier between patient and receptionist, though this can make the privacy of the transaction more difficult to achieve. To be honest, although we see consultations as confidential, most patients do not and are happy to regale the waiting room, family circle or supermarket queue with all their gory details. However, that does not absolve us from the responsibility of catering for patients who do not wish the rest of the waiting room to know about their business. The maintenance of privacy and confidentiality depends more on the skill and tact of the receptionists than the physical surroundings, and they should be trained to be constantly aware of this.

Waiting rooms are often bleak, uncomfortable places and all too often may even be rather dirty. New paint or wallpaper is not expensive and there can be little excuse for grubby walls or peeling paint. Myriads of posters and instructions may cover the walls, whatever their underlying condition. If possible, the temptation to try to communicate with patients in this way should be avoided. A multiplicity of posters looks awful and promotes an institutional aura. Information overload is ineffective and such instructions are likely to be ignored.

Sometimes a practice is stuck with unsatisfactory premises, without hope of making radical alterations, and so has to make the best of a bad job. However, patients should not have to sit around on hard, uncomfortable chairs. Whatever the decor, the chairs should at least be padded and there should be enough of them to go round. With an appointment system, six seats per doctor should cope with waiting patients, relatives and delays; with a non-appointment system more seats than this are needed.

A little thought and effort can go a long way to making the patient more comfortable. Bare walls, for example, can be cheered up considerably by a display of pictures. It can be easy to persuade local art societies to have exhibitions of their members' work in the surgery. Alternatively, local primary or play schools are usually delighted to provide a selection of the childrens' paintings and drawings for display. These are usually very colourful and the children are thrilled to bits knowing that their work is on show to the public.

The trip from the waiting room to the consulting room may cause some problems in a large surgery, particularly with old people who may get lost. Large, clear labels on the rooms help and, if there are any corridors, a system of coloured lights to lead the way to a particular room can be useful. Once the patient gets to the doctor, there should not be a massive deck coming between them. This puts the doctor in an even more dominant position and may inhibit the patient. Seating should be arranged so that the doctor and the patient can face each other without any intervening desk (see p. 189). A pleasant, homely consulting room and a friendly doctor help the patient to relax.

PROVIDING A VARIETY OF SERVICES

Good premises and adequate ancillary help enable the modern general practitioner to provide a wide variety of services. The more that can be provided under one roof, the better. For the patient there is greater convenience and savings in time and travelling expense. For the doctor the provision of good medical care becomes easier and communication with other team members can be enhanced.

Many basic investigations can be carried out in the practice. Practice nurses can be taught to do ESRS, haemoglobins, urine testing, peak flow rates, blood sugars, skin allergy testing and ECGs. They can also collect blood, urine and other samples for transfer to the pathology lab later. If transport is a problem, the samples can often be picked up by the hospital vans which are normally doing rounds in the district.

There should also be no need for the patient to go elsewhere to get children immunised or to have cervical smear tests. Advice about minor ailments or injuries should be readily available from suitably trained practice nurses, and community nurses and health visitors should have a base in the building where patients can contact them directly. In really large premises there may be space to allow people like social workers, registrars of births and deaths, chiropodists and even probation officers to hold sessions for their clients. Cooperative consultants can also arrange to hold sessions in the surgery, which can be convenient for everybody.

With a little imagination and foresight it is possible to give patients a first-class service at little cost to the practice. Heating, lighting and telephone expenses may increase, but even these may be partly reimbursed by the parties concerned, if the responsible authorities are tackled.

As we are self-employed businessmen, services provided should be compatible with earning a reasonable profit each year. Some extra services can pay for themselves by earning extra fees or by retaining patient loyalty and capitation fees. Others will actually cost money which cannot be reimbursed directly. Any new scheme should therefore be carefully assessed to make sure that it is likely to be reasonably cost-effective or so medically effective that the actual costs incurred are worth expending.

Time spent in talking to hospitals or social services staff can be well worth while, because if they can be persuaded that practice ideas will benefit them and the patients, then the help of attached staff may be forthcoming at very little cost.

ADMINISTERING EFFICIENTLY

No matter what range of services are offered to patients, they may not be very happy if they find the staff inefficient or unfriendly. The doctors must give the lead to the rest of the staff. If they always talk as if patients were the enemy, then the staff may reflect this attitude in the way they interact with patients. Receptionists must be mature enough to be able to be friendly and caring while at the same time being quite firm where it is necessary. Their telephone manner and the way they handle patients in the surgery is vital to the success of the practice.

Confidentiality must be maintained by the practice at all times and patients must never feel that inappropriate information about them will ever be disclosed without their permission. Receptionists must learn therefore never to mention names in connection with visits, illnesses or drugs in such a way that bystanders may glean information about the patient concerned.

Day-to-day administration should run as smoothly as possible so that all dealings with the practice can be effected with the minimum of hassle. Telephones are often a source of complaint. There should be enough lines to cope with the peaks and troughs of demand. Patients can get very cross and frustrated if they find lines continually engaged. If the traffic is too heavy, arrangements must be made to even it out or more lines must be installed. Spreading the load can be achieved by asking patients not to phone for repeat prescriptions in the morning when there are normally a lot of requests for appointments or visits.

If more lines are installed, then enough staff should be on duty to deal with the incoming calls. It is just as frustrating to get through to the surgery and then have to wait while the receptionist on the appointments desk deals with three other calls before taking theirs.

Requests for home visits can be a source of friction unless receptionists are well briefed and trained to handle encounters in the way the doctors want them to. Whatever the practice policy is for dealing with visit requests, a key requirement must be that the receptionist is not exposed to hostility while trying to carry out the doctor's orders.

Similarly the repeat prescribing system (see p. 227) must be efficient and allow for easy and convenient access to prescriptions for all those entitled to them. Refusals or changes in medication should be accompanied by a note from the doctor, so that again receptionists are not left coping with patients whose anger and hostility should really be directed at the doctor.

A calm, efficient and friendly atmosphere does a lot to ensure that patients feel welcome and well looked after.

Section 3
Keeping the doctor happy

Introduction

Having considered the needs of patients, we now turn to those of their doctors. Up to a point the interests of both groups are complementary and it seems reasonable to assume that having a happy and satisfied doctor would benefit patients — reasonable, that is, so long as the doctor's happiness has not been gained by a self-centred manipulation of the system invariably to give his or her needs precedence over those of the patients. There has to be an equitable balance between the needs of both parties, with GPs bearing very much in mind the fact that their patients pay handsomely — albeit indirectly through taxation — for any care that they may receive.

THE COST OF CARE

The NHS is not free, far from it. It costs the country about £300 p.a. per person, or over £1000 p.a. per family. Government spending on medical care will exceed £12 888 million in 1983–84, £2923 million of this being the cost of family practitioner services. Whether or not we should be spending more than this is arguable. Certainly we do not spend as much of our Gross National Product on medical care as the US and other Northern European countries, but equally certainly more money will not be forthcoming in the foreseeable future.

There is a very strong case for redeploying our available resources to better advantage before continuing the never-ending cry for more. As doctors we owe two duties to our paymasters: first, to provide as medically effective a service as possible and, second, to provide as cost-effective a service as possible. This latter obligation is most often and most easily overlooked.

GPs make many economic decisions in the course of their work. They control the access of patients to the rest of the health care system and are major allocators of the NHS's resources. Each GP (at 1977 prices) costs the NHS over £100 000 annually; by comparison each consultant costs £500 000 while administration costs, often used by doctors to explain away financial shortages, are only 2.6 percent of total health care expenditure — a figure substantially less than in any other Western country.

It is fair to say that few GPs have any idea of the costs of the services that they allocate or any incentive, other than a general feeling of public-spiritedness, to find out and then practise with some regard to weighing of costs against likely medical benefit. Unfortunately most therapies employed have never been scientifically evaluated. Even when they have, and the best line of practice has been clearly established by study and reasoned argument, the best line is not always adopted. For example, there is clear evidence that for those otitis media cases needing antibiotic therapy a three-day course is clinically as effective as five, seven or ten or more days. Yet, do all or even a majority of GP's prescribe only three days' worth for otitis media?

The volume and costs of ineffective and inefficient procedures could well be huge, yet doctors in the NHS are not highly motivated to practise economically. A professional monopoly by law; rigid adherence to the sacred cow of complete clinical freedom; lack of awareness of the costs of medical actions and the substantial control we exercise over our own working conditions, all conspire to hinder attempts at self-analysis and the exercising of self-control. The fact that exercising such self-control would also be likely to lead to better standards of medical care is an even stronger argument in its favour.

As we are now beginning to sound a bit like a party political broadcast or, even worse, a Grauniad leader, let us end by saying that we believe that the doctor's happiness should not be unthinking but should stem from the firm knowledge that job satisfaction and intellectual stimulation are being achieved while improving performance and benefiting patients — from a realisation that valuable service is being provided and appreciated and that the income engendered represents a worthwhile personal reward for all the effort.

In this section we will outline methods, which can be deployed in any practice, to allow GPs to extract the very best out of professional life.

Choosing a practice

So much of a practitioner's professional wellbeing depends on the nature of the practice that the selection of one's future workplace is of vital importance. All too often the prospective GP concentrates on one or two fairly superficial reasons for choosing a particular practice while ignoring other factors which in the long run may have a much more profound effect.

Choices may be based on a wish to be near to or to get away from family and friends, or on rather romantic self-images of fulfilling the role of friendly rural physician or earnest healer transforming inner-city practice. Though these factors may be important, it is foolish to make decisions without assessing the full implications of working in a practice and its effects on professional and family life.

It is worth bearing in mind that as a doctor grows older his or her ideas and needs, and those of the family, alter. What seems ideal to the 28-year-old with two small children may seem less than perfect ten years later and disastrous once the children have left home. Unlike other professionals, the GP's earning power is relatively stable, and practices cannot be changed without major upheaval and loss of income, as parity has to be painfully regained.

A practice partnership is often likened to a marriage and, whilst divorce is commonplace and relatively cheap in the early years, it can be a crippling financial and emotional burden if it occurs in later life.

WHERE OR WITH WHOM?

Country practice

A small country practice offers the chance of being closely involved with the local community. The GP can get to know all the practice's patients intimately and this encourages a personal, patient-orientated service. Living in the community, the doctor and the family are likely to take part in all the local social and community activities and many patients become friends. Many doctors enjoy this quite intense relationship, though it can sometimes be a strain to maintain a professional stance with patients who are also social acquaintances.

Rural practices normally have small list sizes and high visiting rates which mean a lot of travelling about. Income may be low unless it is boosted by dispensing, which generates a lot of money for very little effort. Because of the distances involved, it is also possible to become isolated professionally and socially, and so before retreating to the depths of the countryside it is wise to determine the wishes of all the family.

Professional isolation is not necessarily alleviated by having one or two partners. If there is any kind of personality clash between them, the feeling of isolation is likely to be enhanced. It is far easier for a large rather than a small group to contain an aberrant partner, though if the partners are compatible and have remained 'switched on', the small country practice can be comfortable, secure and satisfying.

Urban practice

At the other extreme, inner-city practice can offer the challenge of organising care for a large population with high morbidity rates. This is stimulating and rewarding work, provided one can keep up the pace, year after year without any deterioration of standards. The family too will have to cope with inner-city life unless the night work is farmed out to a deputising service and the GP retreats to a home in suburbia or the country.

Bigger groups can offer sophisticated and well-organised care for patients, but if the partners do not work well together the practice is likely to become chaotic and impersonal. Perhaps the ideal practice lies between these extremes and is to be found in 3–6 doctor groups working in small towns.

So, before making a final decision you have to ask yourself many questions including: 'Do I wish to live among my patients and become part of the community?'; 'Can I be a good doctor and a friend to the same people?'; 'Do my spouse and family share my ideas and ideals?'; 'Do I find it easier to cope with social class 1 or social class 4 patients?'

Solo practice

Although single-handed practice is becoming less common, mainly because younger doctors prefer to seek the companionship and mental stimulation that should be available in a group, so many groups are dysfunctional due to personality clashes that some doctors are driven to look for the independence that can be found in solo practice. Others are so socially inept that they cannot get on with their professional peers and so have to work alone. Unfortunately, many of this sub-group of single-handed practitioners cannot relate to their patients either. Although they may quote many reasons for preferring to work alone, there is a nagging doubt that their reasons are really excuses to protect themselves from the scrutiny of their peers. Of course, there is a third sub-group of GPs who are strongly attracted to the concept of giving a highly personal service and who find working by themselves most satisfying.

Without doubt, the price to be paid for practising alone is the real risk of professional isolation and the slow deterioration of standards resulting from a lack of stimulation from others. Though there are strong, sometimes eccentric, individuals who make a great success of single-handed practice, they do seem to be the minority.

REACTIONARY OF REVOLUTIONARY?

At an interview, spend more time looking at the partners than at the premises, area or accounts. Find out as much as you can about the process of policy-making and the practice power structure.

Ask who organised and implemented some of the practice policies. If there are no, or only a few, agreed policies, then the level of intrapractice communication is poor. However this is explained or rationalised — usually by 'we believe in individual freedom' — it really implies that the partners are unable to accept compromises and the fact that they can be wrong. Professionals who are secure and have faith in their own competence can normally discuss their problems and arrive at some logical and acceptable compromise. In a practice where the partners have worked out policies on a variety of clinical and organisational topics, you can be certain that relationships are good.

As any new GP worth his or her salt will want to influence the development of the practice, it is important to find out if the older partners will allow newcomers to propound new theories and try out new ideas. Ask a question like 'Have you ever thought of ...?' where the 'of ...' relates to any part of practice policy or organisation that you have noticed could be changed. If the question is rejected, no matter how politely, without discussion or evaluation, then you may assume that this is likely to be the story of your life if you joined that particular, frustrating, practice.

Ask about the frequency and nature of practice meetings and who does what. This allows identification of the power structure — there always is one. Dominant figures are acceptable, provided decisions are taken in a democratic way and the group can curb the leader when necessary. Frequent meetings indicate a commitment to the development of good communications, a vital point.

Our view is that, though it is important to work in an area and practice that correspond to your ideals, it is even more important to have partners who are friendly, competent and agreeable to change. A partnership in a superficially attractive practice in just the right area could be hell on wheels if the other partners turned out to be medical dinosaurs resisting all new ideas and suggestions. In the long run, greater happiness and job satisfaction might be achieved working in a rather rundown district with a bunch of cheerful, innovative colleagues with flexible personalities.

Getting on with partners

For most doctors the ability to get on at all levels with their partners is the single most important factor in determining whether they are happy or miserable in practice. All other potential partnership or practice problems pale into insignificance beside those thrown up by bitter personality clashes or the internecine warfare generated by dysfunctional relationships.

Of course in many practices the doctors get on well without too much effort, though in a surprising number this is only at the expense of avoiding ever really getting to grips with areas of professional difference. However harmony is achieved, it should not be dependent solely on general feelings of goodwill or the personal characteristics of partners. Getting on with each other in a partnership is something to be worked at. Constructive thought and effort need to be put in and strengthened by policies built into the practice structure.

Mutual respect, consensus decisions and equal reward for equal effort are three of the cornerstones of a good relationship. The fourth and most important is to allow the principle 'Do unto others as you would be done to' to influence partners in all dealings with each other.

MEETING REGULARLY

Good communications are the hallmark of the successful group. All too many partnerships operate as a collection of individuals, meeting only to sort out the most pressing of administrative problems. In these circumstances new ideas are unlikely to be developed or implemented as, stifled by lack of discussion, they are soon abandoned.

Each and every practice should be in a continual state of evolution. This can only be achieved if the partners regularly examine performance and discuss desirable changes. Ossified clinical and organisational habits are characteristic of doctors who have lost enthusiasm for their profession. This may be due to laziness, though it is more likely that the underlying cause is long-term frustration at being unable to achieve ideals in practice.

This highlights another important benefit of regular meetings — the mutual support and encouragement that help doctors to survive the inevitable stresses and strains of everyday general practice. When one makes a clinical mistake or tangles with a particularly difficult patient, it is very reassuring to be able to talk the problem over with someone who understands and is supportive. Sharing feelings, ideas and worries also enables partners to be critical, in a constructive way, about each other's performance. Relationships with each other need to be very secure before criticism can be exchanged freely in this way, but this security is never likely to be achieved unless partners actively pursue the goal of better communications.

Meetings serve three main purposes. First, there is a need for the simple chat and exchange of anecdote which enlivens the day and cements relationships. Then, discussions about problem cases and the venting of anxieties and worries allow the partners to draw on each other's strengths and expertise. Finally, less frequent but more structured, meetings are needed for the formulation of practice policies on clinical and organisational matters.

The only way to make sure that partners actually talk to each other is to arrange the practice timetable so that they are brought together in the same place at the same time with some regularity. These meetings should be given the priority they deserve. If necessary, clinical and other commitments should be reviewed and changed if they interfere with this process. It is all too easy for partners to dash about for weeks on end without actually meeting each other for longer than the few seconds that it takes to pass the time of day. The timetable should be so arranged that at some time during the day all the partners are free of commitments for at least a few minutes. Then they can meet for coffee and a chat. This time together can be extended for at least some of the partners if they can do part of their routine work, e.g. repeat prescriptions, in the same room. They can then both get on with work and chat. The value of this time together should not be underestimated.

Once a week a more formal meeting for case discussions and the sorting out of minor organisational problems should be held. The easiest way to do this is to have a working lunch. Good food helps people to relax, though some formal structure is needed, else there is the danger that all the time will be taken up with anecdotes. A benevolently despotic chairman may be necessary, and it is a good idea to record the more important decisions in a minute book. More weighty matters can be noted for fuller discussion later.

Major policies are best worked out at more formal, longer meetings where subjects can be fully explored. An evening meeting with a meal, rotating loosely to give everyone's spouse a fair share of the cooking, allows business to mix nicely with pleasure. One partner should be responsible for convening these meetings, otherwise it may be many months before someone works up enough steam about a topic actually to organise one. They should be frequent enough to provide some continuity, but not so close together that they begin to pall. Every six to eight weeks seems to be a reasonable compromise, though the exact interval is not as important as the regularity.

Proceedings must be minuted, as memories are notoriously fickle when it comes to recalling decisions at a later date. It may be worth keeping two minute books. One in longhand is kept by the recorder at home and contains a record of everything discussed. A typed copy, with confidential staff matters or other topics for the doctors' eyes only referred back to the private minutes, can be kept in the practice meeting or common room where any partner can refer to them when necessary.

IMPLEMENTING DECISIONS

Once policies are agreed, they have to be implemented. It is all too easy to decide formally on a new course of action and then conveniently forget to implement the decision. As with the management of a troublesome or difficult patient, there may be a tacit collusion between partners actually not to take responsibility for sorting out the problem. To avoid this, a partner or partners should be delegated to operate new policies, and the responsible person should be noted in the minutes. There should be absolutely no confusion about who is meant to do what.

When partners assume responsibility for individual aspects of the practice organisation then everyone, including the ancillary staff, will know exactly whom to approach if something goes wrong or needs to be altered. Of course there cannot be responsibility without the power to implement and follow through policy decisions. A certain amount of freedom to take executive action is necessary to avoid the constant hassle of the partner concerned having to consult other partners before making day-to-day decisions. Responsible partners have to be allowed and trusted to do their best in any particular situation and must not be criticised if their decisions are not always 100 percent correct.

Practice organisation can be conveniently subdivided, with responsibilities allocated to coincide if possible with partners' particular skills and interests. Expertise in handling people, other than in a one-to-one situation, will naturally attract the job of looking after the staff. Training the nurses and receptionists should be the job of somebody who already has some interest in teaching. The business-minded person in the group should get the job of doing the accounts, though an assistant is necessary for this post to avoid confusion in holiday times. Surgery equipment and stock control is another important job, some of which can be delegated to a practice manager or secretary, while overall control remains in the hands of a responsible partner. The bigger the group, the more specialised the organisational roles will be, and the more important it is to have cooperation between partners with clearly defined responsibilities.

Obviously the system of delegation will vary from practice to practice, though an overall plan that is clear to everybody is the only way to get efficiency and a fair distribution of work. If each partner feels involved and appreciated for his or her contribution, then there is less likelihood of anyone feeling that they are not a valuable and respected member of the team. This makes for good relationships.

SHARING INCOME

The principles of equal work for equal pay and absolute honesty in financial dealings within the partnership are fundamental to its good health. The tradition of the senior partner taking the lion's share of the income while doing as little of the work as possible has taken a long time to die out. It was not until the late 1960s and the 1970s that the pressure produced by a shortage of applicants forced the recalcitrant seniors to offer better terms to incoming partners. We hope that the current norm of about three years to full parity will not lengthen in the wake of the glut of young doctors that has just developed. Partners who impose unfair financial terms or workload on a junior must realise that this will be counter-productive in the long term. The young partner is hardly likely to be innovative, enthusiastic or cooperative if he or she has a genuine feeling of resentment at being exploited.

To avoid complications and haggling, we believe that it is fairest and easiest to pool income from all professional activities. This should include everything from seniority payments and vocational training allowances to payments for teaching and outside appointments. Any regular commitment makes a particular doctor less available to the practice. If a factory has to be visited every Friday, then if there is some crisis on a Friday that partner will not be in a position to help the others. Thus the activity, though nominally 'in his or her own time', will still have an effect on practice organisation and inevitably lead to extra work within the practice for the other doctors. Too many junior partners have been pleased to be given an equal share until they find out that they are left minding the shop while the senior partners are out evey afternoon earning extra for their own pockets.

An additional benefit of the pool system is that it discourages partners from working themselves to a frazzle doing evening clinics or nocturnal deputising sessions. A chronically tired partner is hardly likely to be an asset to the practice, which after all should be the overriding concern of all partners and which should take priority over all other activities, rather than the other way round.

The disadvantage of the pool system is that it can be quite difficult to ensure an even distribution of work, and it does produce a positive disincentive to undertake outside activities. This is a mixed blessing, as too many outside activities can adversely affect the delivery of care to the practice patients. However, partners must discuss in some detail what level of extra commitment is compatible with an efficient practice. Outside jobs should be selected for their ability to provide intellectual stimulation and other benefits to the practice, e.g. quicker referrals for practice patients, rather than for the extra income. A small salary divided among partners and then taxed is unlikely to provide much of a financial incentive.

Any activities of one partner will inevitably have some effect on the others. Commitments of any kind must be fully discussed before they are accepted. It is all too easy for one partner to develop an attack of chronic multiple 'committeeitis', leaving the others to cope while he or she is dashing about the country to meetings. Teaching and political activities can stimulate the practice, but the pros and cons have to be weighed up carefully. In the end, a delicate balance has to be reached between the need for individuals to develop particular interests and the service needs of the practice as a whole. A satisfactory compromise will only be reached if partners are genuinely concerned about each other's needs.

Where a practice does decide that partners can earn and keep all or part of their extrapractice professional income, then this is only fair when all partners are governed by the same rules. There must be equal opportunity — though not necessarily equal ability — to pursue remunerative activities. The details of the business relationship should be clearly written into the partnership agreement.

HAVING A PROPER AGREEMENT

In a happy·group there should be little need ever to refer to a written partnership agreement, other than for updating if conditions within the partnership change. However, it is still vital for every practice to have a carefully thought-out contract to provide an unbiased reference source for the resolution of any potentially serious partnership disagreements or arguments.

Among other things, the agreement should spell out in detail:

1. The division of practice income among the partners.
2. The right of any partner to inspect the practice accounts at any time.
3. Each partner's entitlement to sick leave, study leave and holidays.
4. The disposition of income from extrapractice commitments and the agreement necessary among partners before such commitments are taken on.
5. The age at which partners must retire and other circumstances under which they might be deemed to have left the partnership.
6. Where partners may live.
7. What majorities are needed for decisions to be made and how arbitration will be effected in the event of irreconcilable differences.

There are many other important points, and advice should be taken from the BMA's Personal Services Bureau or solicitors before any agreement is finalised.

Though it is hard to imagine any modern practice effecting its business without a written agreement, apparently only 50 percent of practices actually have such agreements. For the others we can only strongly advise that a specimen agreement, plus guidelines for what should be covered by it, is obtained from the BMA and that a few practice meetings are set aside to hammer out a working practical agreement purpose-designed to reflect the practice's individual needs.

INTERACTING SOCIALLY

Some social contact among partners and their families helps to cement relationships and friendships, though it is not at all necessary to live in each other's pockets. Practice dinners and the odd party allow the spouses to meet and enable the partners to relax without discussing business. These semi-official events are not a substitute for, but a supplement to, individual friendships and serve to keep all partners and spouses in amiable contact. In our practice we have three practice (partnership) functions a year and take turns to do the organising.

While social contacts are necessary, spouses should not feel that they are obliged to maintain an excessive 'friendship' with each other. Forced involvement with one another and with the workings of the practice can lead to personality clashes and the inevitable involvement of the partners themselves. When spouses voice their own feelings about practice affairs too loudly, feathers may be ruffled. Friendships should develop naturally or not at all.

Limited social contact means that social niceties can be easily maintained, while oversocialising, which might cause friction, is avoided.

Well-organised communications and a watertight contract will avail nothing without tolerance. We must be able to tolerate different political or religious views as well as each other's quirks of personality. Any partner should be able to disagree without losing respect.

There is also a need to be realistic about each other's strengths and weaknesses. Strengths should be encouraged and developed. Weaknesses should not be ignored. They should be discussed kindly when appropriate, with support offered when necessary. Doctors are very wary about this sort of interaction, but avoiding the problem does not help anybody. The partnership group can be therapeutic, though one must be careful not to get too intense about this. Help should be sought from outside if a particular partner's problems seem too complex to be solved internally.

Maintaining standards

Continuing job satisfaction depends to a large degree on the achievement of high standards of practice for patients who appreciate the service. In recent years, general practitioners have become far more aware of their academic abilities and have taken increasing pride in realising, rather than just paying lip service to, high standards of care.

This process involves the GP in keeping up to date with the latest practice and medical developments; keeping good records to provide a wealth of information and insight into the what and how of the practice's activities; and being prepared and able to audit work patterns and, if necessary, to modify them.

STAYING SWITCHED ON

Above all, staying switched on is an attitude of mind that is of value to the doctor, whatever the circumstances. An open and enquiring mind is prepared to question, discuss and learn anywhere and any time. It is also prepared to stimulate and be stimulated by others, both inside and outside the practice.

Though the right mental attitude is fundamental, it has to be allied to self-discipline and effort, if the knowledge and skills gained are going to be practically applied to the benefit of others. Knowledge without application is just as useless, though not as dangerous, as application without knowledge.

Self-education

Once vocational training is finished, further educational opportunities are provided by clinical tutors in postgraduate centres and meetings organised by the RCGP and other bodies. No-one, apart from the individual concerned and perhaps his or her partners, can make a doctor keep up to date. Further education must be seen as desirable in its own right, and a partnership should actively strive to provide an environment which will stimulate this activity.

Unfortunately, no-one can force their attentions on a closed or unreceptive mind. Two main areas to consider are:

1. *Practice literature* Every GP should cultivate the self-discipline necessary to read regularly and comprehensively at least two of the many excellent journals that clamour for our attention. The *BMJ* and a review journal such as *Update* would fill the bill admirably, though the useful knowledge and practical tips to be gained from regular, albeit selective, reading of weekly medical newspapers such as *Pulse, General Practitioner* or *Doctor* should not be underestimated.

Good articles should be abstracted and filed — it requires little effort to devise an individual system for doing this — to provide a personal reference system for future learning, research, writing or what have you. A good personal and practice library, selected from the increasing number of high-quality practice-relevant books becoming available, is also a must for broadening horizons and providing a secure knowledge base from which to strike out.

After reading may come writing, which has its own learning disciplines and rewards.

2. *Postgraduate education* For too long this potentially useful source of educational activity has been in the hands of consultants who have taken a very narrow view of medicine and have made arbitrary, and wrong, decisions about what general practitioners ought to be taught. The result has been didactic lectures and courses geared to the concepts of hospital medicine and guaranteed to stultify all but the dullest intellects.

While there is still a place for the formal lecture, it has become apparent that there are other more effective ways of learning. General practitioners have a lot that they can teach each other, and discussion in small groups enables them to explore their problems and to formulate answers. This format is particularly useful for looking at the delivery of medical care. Subjects for discussion can include the use of appointment systems, the value of screening programmes, the long-term care of diabetics.

Large practices can sustain their own groups, but smaller practices need to join up with others for this purpose. This can be done through the local postgraduate centre or can be organised by the practice concerned. If the local clinical tutor provides the same boring old lectures year after year, then it behoves the local GPs to ask for a new approach or to organise it themselves.

In addition to local courses, there is an extensive choice of more exotic fare on offer through agencies such as the British Postgraduate Medical Federation. A complete change of scene for a few days each year to learn what others think and do can be most stimulating. Every practice should consider allowing each partner a week's study leave a year. Clearly, to be of benefit this time should only be used for bona fide learning and not for other more nefarious activities. It is an unusual partner, no matter how bored with self-education exercises otherwise, who will not avail himself or herself of this facility. Once there, whatever the motivation, some benefit will accrue.

Teaching and learning

Any practice that is genuinely interested in maintaining high standards should consider being involved in either undergraduate or postgraduate teaching. The presence of a student or trainee acts as a spur, stimulating activities and development that might otherwise have been neglected. Having to explain one's actions and policies to a young colleague with a keen and critical mind forces clear thought about what is being done. The learning process is, of course, a two-way affair, and trainees can be a constant source of new ideas and knowledge.

For practices which wish to involve themselves in training new GPs, it is worth noting that trainer selection committees are becoming ever more stringent in the application of their criteria. The potential training practice therefore has to demonstrate that it is well organised; has a high standard of medicine; and has the time, the expertise, the enthusiasm and the required standard of records. These requirements force the practice to look at itself critically and to make any necessary changes. This process can provide a very useful tool and be used by a forward-looking partner to influence more reactionary colleagues. Through the carrots of money and an extra pair of hands, yardsticks of good practice can be applied and change given impetus and direction. The trainer too will be given added stimulus from discussion and argument at trainers' workshops and the local Vocational Training Course.

There are many other groups apart from trainees and medical students who need teaching and training. General practitioners can and should be involved in health education, first-aid classes, receptionist training and the education of nurses, health visitors and other ancillary staff attached to the practice.

Teaching of any kind is a stimulating activity and is well worthwhile. It need not be confined to small audiences, as the growth of local radio and the media's general preoccupation with medical matters allows interested doctors to communicate with the public at large. The advice given should be accurate and up to date and, if it upsets the sensitivities of less-aware colleagues, then it is they rather than the communicator who should look to their laurels.

Research

It is fair to say that the large majority of GPs, including us, have little interest in research unless it is of an obviously practical nature. We see this as one of our major deficiencies, as there is so much useful work crying out to be done in practice. For example in defining the natural history of many disorders and to determine their correct/best management.

However, most GPs are happy to help others with their research, and many trials have only succeeded because of practice cooperation. Helping others with genuine research, not drug companies with spurious 'money for putting your patients on Brand X for six months' (and hopefully leaving them on for ever more) type trials, is a worthy and interesting activity.

Effecting purely practice-based research may also be exciting but does require individuals of a certain stamp. Well-organised practices and practitioners can provide the soil from which much valid observation may spring.

The College

In recent years membership of the Royal College of General Practitioners has risen rapidly, because of rather than in spite of the MRCGP examination, to over 10 000. For most young doctor the College is the exam, and the exam is becoming recognised as being as worthwhile and valuable as any other membership qualification. However, even among young doctors there are ambivalent feelings towards the College, which many see as elitist with a leadership getting ever more out of touch with the mainstream of general practice.

Unbiased observers, particularly those who are old enough to remember the phenomenal changes that have taken place in the last twenty years, appreciate that the College has been the main driving force behind much of the change. Whatever one thinks about the present attitudes and behaviour of the leadership, it seems a shame that so few new members take an active part in formulating policy. As in any big organisation, democracy will only work if the constituents participate in the process.

General practice does need an organisation that is dedicated to improving the standards of patient care and to providing a forum for the exchange of ideas. The College does just this, both at local and national level. Though its main concerns are education and research, it is increasingly looked on by government as the most respectable, and most influential, voice speaking for general practice. However unfair this may appear to those who feel their standards of practice owe nothing to the College, this is reality. Those wishing to have their say in the development of modern practice would be well advised to magnify their voices through the College megaphone rather than cry in the wilderness.

For active members prepared to contribute, the rewards, educational and otherwise, make the effort well worthwhile.

KEEPING WORTHWHILE RECORDS

Many a good practice is let down by the standard of its record keeping. Achieving worthwhile records (see p. 207) is a somewhat boring, repetitive and time consuming activity and so it is often accorded a low level of priority. Good records are an essential aid to good practice and fulfil a variety of functions.

The value of good records

1. An accurate aide-memoire No matter how good our memories may be, we cannot hope to remember all the details about even the most familiar patient. Many doctors love to kid themselves about their comprehensive knowledge of their patients, but a careful search of any record envelope will be virtually guaranteed to produce some important piece of information that has been forgotten.

At most, if not all, consultations the doctor needs to have easy and relevant access to the past medical history, social history and current investigations, drugs and management. In group practices where patients may be seen by different doctors, accurate, legible notes are even more important. Deficient notes may give rise to dangerous confusion and duplication of effort, not to mention the possible legal consequences.

Poor records often compromise what could otherwise be a reasonable defence against a claim of negligence. Clear, precise notes might one day save your professional life.

2. *An aid to planned care* Standards of care can be enhanced by the use of a carefully planned record system. Special, practice-designed, flow-charts can facilitate the regular monitoring of long-term problems such as diabetes or hypertension. The card design (see p. 215) standardises the doctor's responses and reminds/forces the doctor to carry out the agreed procedures. No-one feels easy not taking a BP, for example, when the card has a square labelled BP waiting to be filled in.

The best-known and most widely accepted card of this nature is the antenatal cooperation card. While it serves some function as a method of communication, it also standardises antenatal care by specifying which checks are to be done and when.

3. *The basis for a recall system* A recall system is a safeguard for patients with a disease that needs periodic assessment. The names of identified patients are entered into a disease register which the secretary refers to, once every 6–12 months, then to check the notes of all those listed to ensure that they have attended for follow-up. Defaulters can be sent a letter to remind them to attend. Any practice without some sort of recall system will have some patients with diseases like hypertension, diabetes, myxoedema who have stopped attending or taking their medication, because they feel well and do not wish to bother the doctor.

A morbidity index, linked to the recall register, is another waay to keep track of patients, and also allows audit of the practice's management of that disease; identification of cases for research or teaching; and recall of patients if, for example, a new treatment might be of benefit to them.

Achieving better records

Having appreciated that good records are not merely desirable but essential to improve standards of care, GPs wishing to bring their systems up to date must also appreciate the amount of sheer hard work that is going to be involved. Virtually every patient envelope is going to have remedial surgery to trim off surplus information and to organise the rest into an easily accessible and retrievable form.

While this effort goes on — and it will take years rather than months — old habits must be changed so that a new generation of rubbish-filled cards are not being produced in the meantime. Let us look at the matter logically:

1. A4 or Lloyd-George? The Lloyd-George envelope is small, with such little room for hospital letters and reports that it severely restricts the total amount of information that can be retained. This need not be a disadvantage, as the useful information that needs to be retained for any patient is small. Also, if the record is thinner and the relevant information more clearly presented then it is more likely that this information is actually going to be useful to the doctor.

For a long time, A4 records were regarded as the panacea for all record-keeping ills, despite the horrendous cost in time and money that conversion to them would require. They take up more than three times the room that conventional records do, and so the practice using them needs increased storage space.

The main argument against them is that merely increasing the size of the file has little effect on the quality of the contents. You only have to look at the average bulky hospital record file to realise that size and efficiency are not one and the same thing. The keeper of a totally disorganised Lloyd-George envelope will only produce a totally disorganised A4 record, unless some dramatic conversion has taken place in the meantime.

2. Careful note-taking When rushed, most GPs would rather spend an extra half a minute with the patient than writing notes, so to be realistic, notes must be kept as short as possible. Clarity and brevity also aid greatly in the retrieval of information, particularly if important features such as the diagnosis or investigations are highlighted in some way, e.g. by being written or ringed in red or green (Fig. 3.1).

Whether all partners use, or not, depending on their proclivities, some variant of the SHIT or SOAP (Subjective, Objective, Assessment, Plan) systems does not matter so long as a brief record is made of each consultation covering: the problem presented; important positive and negative verbal and physical findings; description of condition or diagnosis; and management plan. Needless to say, this should be legible, and some unfortunate doctors may find this the most difficult hurdle.

3. Contents into date order A fundamental aspect of record-keeping is the need to have the contents in some sort of date order. Nothing is more frustrating than having to look through a mass of cards and letters that are in a hopeless jumble. Under these circumstances, there is a good chance of important information being missed.

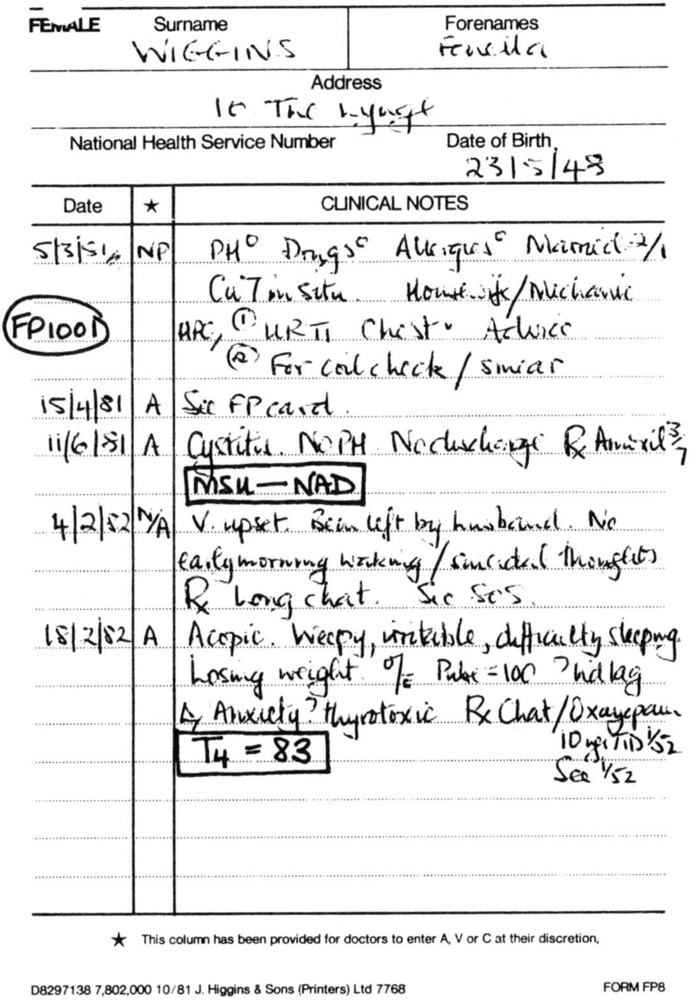

FEMALE Surname WIGGINS | Forenames Fenella

Address
10 The ...

National Health Service Number | Date of Birth 23/5/48

Date	★	CLINICAL NOTES
5/3/81	NP	PH° Drugs° Allergies° Married 2/1 Cu7 in situ. Housewife/Mechanic
(FP1001)		HRC, ① URTI Chest ✓ Advice ② For coil check / smear
15/4/81	A	See FP card.
11/6/81	A	Cystitis. No PH No discharge Rx Amoxil 3/7 MSU — NAD
4/2/82	N/A	V. upset. Been left by husband. No early morning waking / suicidal thoughts Rx Long chat. See SOS.
18/2/82	A	Acopic. Weepy, irritable, difficulty sleeping. Losing weight. O/E Pulse = 100 ? lid lag Δ Anxiety ? thyrotoxic Rx Chat/Oxazepam 10 mg TID 1/52 See 1/52 T4 = 83

★ This column has been provided for doctors to enter A, V or C at their discretion.

D8297138 7,802,000 10/81 J. Higgins & Sons (Printers) Ltd 7768 FORM FP8

Fig. 3.1 Clear, legible notes are well worth achieving.

Sorting out a cabinet full of disorganised records is a daunting task, but putting things into date order and trimming letters to size is not skilled work. Most practices do not employ their full ration of ancillary staff, so getting a youngster in to do the job is not very expensive, particularly as 70 percent of the cost is reimbursable. If you already have a full staffing ratio, a word with the local FPC administrator will often result in permission to employ extra staff, temporarily, to upgrade records or to compile an age–sex register.

All the practice staff should be taught to be conscious of the need for good records. When anybody spots a tatty envelope or a set of notes that are too bulky or disorganised, they should take the initiative and pass the cards on to whoever is responsible for the appropriate action. This may just be for making out a new envelope, though it could also mean putting the cards on the doctor's desk with a polite suggestion that perhaps this record could do with a summary. If the doctors, secretaries and receptionists all egg each other on to improve the records, then steady progress is possible.

The effort is well worthwhile and a box full of clean, tidy, slim and useful records at the start of a surgery is quite a morale-booster.

4. *Summarising and filleting* Ideally, every record should contain a summary of all important medical events and social conditions, on an easily identified summary card (Fig. 3.2) (see also p. 210). This card should be a distinct colour and is of immense help in the consultation, obviating the need to plough through the cards and hospital letters looking for information while trying to talk or listen to the patient. A clear summary also avoids the possibility of overlooking some important detail.

Once again we have to be realistic. Summarising notes is an immense task and will normally take several years of considerable effort. Start your summarising campaign by tackling the 'fat' envelopes. You will learn a lot about your patients in the process, and it will also give you the opportunity to get rid of a mass of unnecessary material. Many doctors seem to be very worried about the legal implications of throwing anything away. The answer is of course that one has to be reasonably selective, but there can be no case for keeping masses of follow-up letters or old investigation reports.

Some longer and more important letters can be retained but even most of them can be summarised and thrown away. If a note is kept of the hospital and the reference number one can always get back to the original record in the unlikely event of any legal or other query. Remember FPCs only keep records of dead patients for 3 years before completely destroying them.

Virtually all fat envelopes can be reduced to a size where the contents will fit in a non gusseted envelope. This makes them look far less intimidating and will actually make them more useful. It is also amazing how a thin envelope changes the doctor's perception of the patient and lessens the likelihood of premature judgments being made.

In some practices medical secretaries have been taught to do summaries. While this is practical, it does need a lot of training and the results have to be monitored from time to time. A simpler

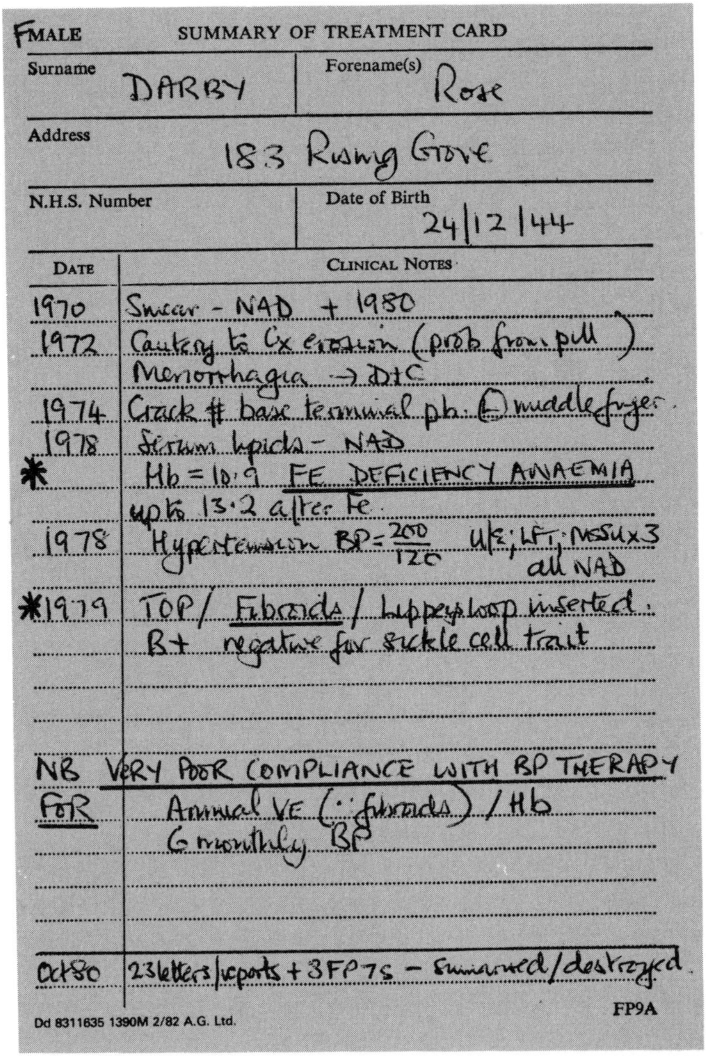

FMALE SUMMARY OF TREATMENT CARD

Surname: DARBY — Forename(s): Rose

Address: 183 Rising Grove

N.H.S. Number: — Date of Birth: 24/12/44

DATE	CLINICAL NOTES
1970	Smear - NAD + 1980
1972	Cautery to Cx erosion (prob from pill)
	Menorrhagia → D+C
1974	Crack # base terminal ph. (L) middle finger.
1978	Serum lipids - NAD
*	Hb = 10.9 FE DEFICIENCY ANAEMIA
	up to 13.2 after Fe.
1978	Hypertension BP = 200/120 U/E; LFT; MSU x3 all NAD
*1979	TOP / Fibroids / Lippes loop inserted.
	B+ negative for sickle cell trait
NB	VERY POOR COMPLIANCE WITH BP THERAPY
FOR	Annual VE (∵ fibroids) / Hb
	6 monthly BP
Oct 80	23 letters/reports + 3 FP7s - summarised/destroyed

Dd 8311635 1390M 2/82 A.G. Ltd. FP9A

Fig. 3.2 The summary card can be used to cue the doctor into providing good care. Any partner seeing the patient can easily assimilate the relevant information.

method is for the doctor to scan the letters and to mark them with a code indicating which ones should be destroyed, which ones need summarising and which ones have to be kept in their entirety. With some training a medical secretary can soon sort out what information is important in a letter, but this process can be aided by the doctor marking relevant passages with a felt-tip pen.

5. *The age-sex register* This register (see p. 220) can enhance the usefulness of a practice's records. Popularised by the College, and suspected purely of being a requirement for recognition of a training practice, many were set up after much effort and anguish, yet were never subsequently used. Before spending time and money, the practice should be clear about what the register is to be used for when it is completed.

The commonest use is to keep track of under-5s so that appropriate developmental surveillance and immunisation is carried out. Even if computer printouts are available, they are not 100 percent reliable and do not help the practice to identify immunised youngsters joining the practice. Other potential preventative uses include the identification of teenage girls in need of rubella vaccination; 20–60-year-old women in need of cervical smear tests; over-70-year-olds who have not been seen during the last year or so.

The age–sex register is an essential tool for almost any form of epidemiological research in general practice. The age–sex structure of practice populations vary so much that facts and figures about any group of patients are meaningless unless they can be related to an accurate picture of the overall age-sex structure of the actual practice population at risk.

Computers

The role of microcomputers (see p. 231) in general-practice record-keeping is currently being evaluated. Initially hailed as the answer to all our recording problems, some disasters have led to more sober appraisal. No matter how powerful the computer or how sophisticated the software, the usefulness and effectiveness will depend entirely on the quality of the information fed in. Potential users consistently underestimate the tremendous amount of hard work that is involved in putting even the most basic details about patients into the system.

Before seriously thinking about buying a system, a practice should define exactly what it is doing badly and then marry this information up with what a computer can do to see whether it might be an appropriate means of solving the problems. The practice without any registers yet possessing a mass of disorganised records must not imagine that a computer is suddenly going to transform the scene. Only hard work will.

The patient registration file is common to all systems. This is a rather detailed age–sex register which, according to the size of the system, can be expanded to contain a variety of details of previous medical and social problems. The computer's main advantage over manual systems is the speed at which this information can then be located and printed out. It can carry out all the functions of a manual age–sex register, but can also provide accurate summaries for insurance reports or for the practitioner at the start of a surgery session.

Most of the GP computer systems on offer can provide some search and analysis facilities. Every practice possesses an immense amount of medical data which, if analysed properly, could provide new facts about epidemiology and the interrelationship of diseases, social conditions and treatment. This opens up a number of possibilities for research.

Repeat prescribing is the only field where a computer may actually reduce a doctor's workload. Once the patient's medication details are entered, repeat prescriptions can be produced rapidly and safely. There are usually built-in safeguards to prevent patients getting drugs for too long without being seen, and some systems also have drug interaction warnings.

Additional software modules can provide accountancy and word processing facilities.

The ultimate aim of most computer buffs is to be able to use a terminal in the consulting room to gain access to the patient's records and to enter new information during the consultation. The difficulty is speed of input. If it takes too long to type in the details, then it is a non-starter in the context of the GP consultation. Most systems record problems in code, and the task of coding and then typing in is too tedious. However, one company is developing a system that has the coding already built in, and all the operator has to do is to type in the first few letters of the diagnosis or the problem. This has great potential, as it takes only a few seconds, and we may yet see the day when every GP has a VDU on the desk.

INDULGING IN AUDIT

Though small practices in particular will benefit from discussions with others, there is still plenty of scope in any practice for internal education and the study of practice activities (see p. 241). Work being done needs to be regularly analysed and then policies to determine the appropriate medical responses need to be devised.

Simple procedures

There are many simple ways of gaining useful information, and practice staff should collect and collate background statistics routinely. Figures for the number of patients seen or visited can be converted into doctor or practice consultation and visiting rates. These rates can be compared with other practices' figures or can be used to monitor workload changes within the practice itself.

Figures for the number of patients per doctor, numbers of patients over 65 and 75, numbers registered for contraceptive care are provided quarterly by the FPC. They can be supplemented by the practice's own figures for vaccinations performed, smears taken, X-rays ordered, lab tests sent off, referrals to hospitals made and so on to provide a clear picture of at least part off what is being done. If the number of vaccinations or smears effected is far less than the population at risk would benefit from, then the questions 'Why?' and 'What should we do about it?' should be posed.

From time to time it is useful to examine in more detail exactly what the doctors are doing. Simple forms can be designed to record the nature and outcome of each consultation. Data can be collected about age, sex, diagnosis, acute or chronic case, patient or doctor initiated consultation, and type of prescription given, if any. This will give an insight into recall rates and prescribing habits, both of which have important implications. One hundred consecutive patients recorded and analysed for each partner will provide a fund of information and an entertaining hour or two of discussion.

The figures may show that one partner has a high recall rate and so clogs up his or her appointments with work the other partners feel able to manage more confidently, or that another partner sees far more young women for contraception than anyone else. Objective analysis of prescribing habits, which can also be gained from the Pricing Bureau, or by keeping carbon copies of all prescriptions issued for 2–3 weeks, often reveals unsuspected problems and differences. Does the partner who boasts about a low hypnotic prescribing rate really practise what he or she preaches? Once the facts are known they can be discussed.

Similarly, an audit of referral letters or number and type of investigations ordered can yield useful information. Widely divergent habits can be explored and common policies formulated. For example, should all women with missed periods have pregnancy tests; when should MSUs be taken; when, if at all, should boils or impetigo lesions be swabbed; do all diabetics need to be referred to hospital; what are the indications for referring children with suspected glue ear?

This type of audit is easy to implement and only needs to be carried out occasionally to monitor what is going on. Why then is it done so infrequently in practice? Lack of time is no excuse, as it only takes about five seconds to fill in a data collection sheet after a patient has left the consulting room. The hesitation is due to the fact that we have not been trained to expect audit and, if anything, we have been taught to regard individual clinical judgment as of paramount importance. Insecurity and fear of criticism is really behind the defensiveness, as well as the force of established practice which makes it necessary for the established GP to make a conscious effort to deviate from the habits of a professional lifetime.

Analysing consultations

Another aspect of audit that is little used, except in a few teaching practices, is the recording and analysis of consultations. Hearing yourself consult on tape or, better still, seeing yourself on video can be a salutary and thought-provoking experience.

Exchanging tapes with another doctor is a far less threatening way of observing behaviour and far more natural than having another doctor sitting in on a consultation. Mutual analysis of tapes can pick up aberrant behaviour which may be decreasing the effectiveness of the consultation. Doctors are often quite unaware of their odd habits and their possible effects on patients. Constructive criticism can help to improve consultation techniques.

This activity is likely to be even more productive if one or more partners have been on a course specifically dealing with consultation analysis.

Supporting each other

Audit activities within the practice need not be threatening at all. If everybody has to undergo the same process and if the discussions are tactful and supportive, the experience can be a great help. Far from being a threat, the support can make all the difference to the partner who is trying to change a particular type of behaviour. For instance, a particular doctor may be aware that too many prescriptions are being given for hypnotics, but he or she may find it difficult to resist importuning patients. Identification of the problem and open discussion will strengthen resolve, while strategies learned from the others can be deployed. The fact that performance is likely to be analysed again in the not too distant future provides the motivation to persist with one's efforts.

Devising protocols

A beneficial consequence of audit is that it forces judgments about what constitutes good rather than bad medical care. If these judgments are being made, then it is as well for partners to sit down and make them together so that practical policies can be worked out to apply the judgments to clinical practice (see p. 237).

To formulate a practice policy it helps if one partner, preferably with a special interest in the subject, reviews the literature to ensure that the knowledge on which decisions are going to be made is up to date. Possible lines of action then have to be discussed to lead to a group decision based on fact and logic, rather than on the whim of a local consultant or a persuasive drug rep.

The policy then has to be implemented by all partners who, perhaps for the first time, will be giving consistent advice to all their patients. Neighbours with the same complaint will no longer have to wonder why one was given tablets while the other was told that nothing was necessary.

Once a practice has decided the principle of having clinical protocols, a simple topic should be chosen for the first attempt. In our group we tackled diarrhoea and decided that no drugs were to be prescribed at all, except for a chronic problem such as colitis or where acute enteritis was making an old person incontinent. Instead, the partners were to confine themselves to giving detailed advice about fluid replacement, particularly in children.

It was quite easy to monitor progress and it was remarkable how soon patients got to know that no prescription would be forthcoming. Though we encouraged parents to bring children for examination, the number of consultations for mild enteritis fell. Encouraged by this, we went on to formulate policies for respiratory infections, diabetes, hypertension, the Pill, antenatal care, the use of hypnotics and many others. Some policies are easier to implement than others, but in every case the attempt has been well worthwhile.

The difficulties we experienced changing from prescribing to non-prescribing for certain minor conditions were certainly eased by the fact that we are a near-monopoly supplier of care. Doctors in more competitive situations may find persuasion tougher. However, our advantage in this respect was balanced by the disadvantage of having a high turnover within our practice population. This means that every year nearly 2500 of our educated patients are replaced by pupils from other schools. We then have the initial extra effort of going through the whole process time and again with different patients.

The multiple audit activities we describe sound rather frenetic and intimidating. Used episodically, they take up very little time and should not be threatening.

Consulting comfortably

To consult comfortably, GPs must be confident in their medical knowledge; assured that the rest of the practice is functioning smoothly while they work; at ease physically; and also psychologically at ease, prepared to deal with any patient or presenting problem.
Broadly speaking, physical and psychological factors have to be considered.

PROMOTING PHYSICAL COMFORT

General practittioners, like anyone else, perform more efficiently in comfortable and attractive surroundings. The consulting room should be a pleasant and easy place to work in, though the furnishings and decor will reflect the personality of the occupant.
It is vital to make the room welcoming to patients, and pictures, plants and other decorations can be used to brighten up even the most austere of settings. A toy or two for the children may also be helpful.
Whether the room itself should be very tidy or not is debatable. Cleanliness is expected, but a too clean and tidy room may be intimidating. An untidy or lived-in room may be less threatening, especially to patients whose children go on the demolition trail, but if it is too much of a mess the patient may doubt the doctor's ability to organise even simple matters.

Calling patients

Though some doctors personally collect their next patient from the waiting room, most prefer to control events while remaining seated. As patients come in and out on average every 5–6 minutes, an efficient call system is necessary to avoid too much waiting time.

A commonly used system, which works well, involves the doctor in pressing a button to activate a buzzer or light or both in the reception area. There, the receptionist either calls the patient and directs him or her to the doctor, or the doctor's name lit up itself alerts the next patient. Other doctors use intercom systems to call patients directly from the waiting room. Depending on the acoustics, this can make the waiting room noisy and a bit like a railway station.

However the patient is called, the doctor should be able to use the few seconds' grace between patients to scan the patient's envelope and notes, both to refresh the memory and to ascertain if any screening procedures should be performed or recommended.

The surgery layout

Whatever else the surgery layout may dictate, the patient should not have to face the doctor across the physical and psychological barrier of a desk (see p. 189). This increases the doctor's power and control and may well inhibit insecure patients from saying all that should be said. The physical barrier is also inhibiting to the doctor as it prevents easy observation of lumps, bumps or rashes and stops spontaneous comforting or encouraging contact. A hand on an arm or hand can help a distressed patient far more than words and can ease the pain of some traumatic experiences.

A chair beside the desk is best, and the doctor's chair should be on wheels, so that it can be moved around as necessary: towards the patient when encouragement is needed and away when the interchange is to be drawn to a close. A right-handed doctor should have the patient on the right, and vice versa. If possible, light from a window should fall on the patient, though this should never be a strong light coming from behind the doctor, as this will make him or her appear as an anonymous silhouette.

Examining patients

There is much debate about whether or not the examination couch should be in the consulting room or in an examination room. A compromise is probably best, with both a couch in the consulting room and easy access to another room with a couch where patients can undress at leisure.

Many examinations in general practice do not need the patient to be fully undressed, and if they can just hop up onto a couch much time will be saved. However, a couch in a room should be curtained off. Women patients who need a breast or vaginal examination can undress quite quickly and do not need to be shunted off to another room, though they do need to be able to undress in privacy. A remarkable number of doctors seem to think that all women can perform a striptease in the consulting room without embarrassment, just because they are with a doctor. The fact that they do not complain is no indication of their feelings, as they may well think that they are being foolish. We think that it is common courtesy to give privacy to someone undressing or dressing. The actual examination is far less embarrassing.

Patients needing a longer examination or a lengthy peeling-off of corsets and several layers of underwear need a separate room. An examination room *per se* is useless if it is not adequately sound-proofed. The GP should be able to see another patient while the first is undressing, but this is impossible if the patient in the examination room can hear all that is going on. As doors are almost impossible to sound-proof, there should not be a connecting door between the consulting room and the examination room.

By using a consulting room with a couch, a spare consulting room can be used while a slow undresser disrobes in the original room. This allows consultations to be completed in the room where the patient first presented, though it does involve the doctor in some moving about.

While common courtesy demands that a patient have privacy to undress, the need for a chaperone is less certain. GPs are divided on this issue. Some, and no doubt the Defence Societies as well, would argue that it is foolish for a male doctor to examine a woman unchaperoned, because of the possibility of being accused of indecent assault.

On the other hand, always to use a chaperone would pose administrative and organisational problems which would make the smooth running of a surgery wellnigh impossible. Chaperones therefore need to be used selectively — just how selectively will depend on the circumstances and the feelings of the doctor.

In a busy surgery where there are many people within easy screaming range it is reasonable to reserve the use of chaperones to high-risk patients, e.g. known hysterics, shy young maidens. Where the patient is being asked to return for a pelvic examination after a period or for a routine smear, she can be asked to bring a friend with her, if she so wishes.

Being discriminating about the use of chaperones does not mean taking unnecessary risks. No woman should be intimately examined if there is no-one else close by or if there are any doubts about her stability. Too many trusting, naive doctors have had the unpleasant experience of being unjustifiably accused of indecent assault.

Equipment

The amount of equipment in a room depends on personal working habits, the amount of routine work normally delegated to the practice nurse and the availability of other areas, e.g. a treatment room for carrying out some procedures.

Any room should have everything necessary for basic examinations, including various sizes of vaginal speculae, and facilities for sterilising them if a central autoclave is not available; proctoscopes; ophthalmoscope/oroscope; sphygmomanometer, possibly with an extra one attached to the wall over the couch; and a peak flow meter. These and other necessities should be stored neatly but within easy reach.

A storage unit round the wash-hand basin provides a handy storage facility, as does a small trolley. Desk or shelf storage units are also needed for forms and stationery.

REMAINING PSYCHOLOGICALLY AT EASE

For effective consultation, the doctor's full attention should be focussed on the patient. Whatever time is actually available, patients should feel that a reasonably unhurried and thoughtful consideration has been given to their problems.

To be able to concentrate in this way, the doctor has to consult without distraction. A secure knowledge base and the ability to cope with difficult people helps prevent internal turmoil interfering too much with thought processes. Similarly, loss of concentration caused by interruptions or the feelings of pressure engendered by running well behind appointment times have to be prevented or coped with.

Let us look at some of these areas in more detail.

Working without interruptions

A telephone in the consulting room is essential, but must be used with discretion. Its imperious tones can seriously disrupt a consultation, and more than one call coming through during a patient's 5–6 minutes makes a mockery of the whole proceedings.

Staff should be trained to interrupt a consultation in person or by phone only when it is really necessary. Colleagues and family, who should know when not to call, should probably be put straight through, though even they could leave a number with the promise that they would be called back as soon as the consultation finished.

Good practice organisation with well-trained staff will minimise this problem. Having a duty doctor who is free to deal with all medical and other emergencies while the rest of the partners consult is also very helpful.

Pacing the consultation

Average consultation lengths may vary considerably from doctor to doctor. At first sight it would seem obvious that the longer the time given to each patient, then the better the standard of care. This is too simple a conclusion to draw about such a complex activity.

A rapid turnover of patients may indicate either a poor doctor fobbing off patients with inappropriate prescriptions or referrals, or a good doctor consulting appropriately with better-than-average organisational and communication skills. Equally, a slow turnover of patients may indicate a poor doctor wasting time in truly idle chatter or non-productive efforts, or a good doctor so well organised and willing to sort out problems effectively that his or her surgery has become overloaded with new patients requiring time-consuming, careful evaluation.

So one partner may happily see twelve patients an hour, having packed the surgery with patients trained to attend repeatedly with trivial illnesses, to attend over-frequently for check-ups of chronic conditions or to attend for unnecessary follow-ups. Another may only see six to eight patients an hour while indulging in non-productive medical procedures and social niceties. The third may be the only one truly troubleshooting, seeing ten patients an hour but attracting all those who have realised how ineffective the other doctors really are.

In the three examples quoted all the partners may in fact over-run their appointment times: the first because someone may present with a problem that cannot be resolved by merely giving another five-minute appointment for the following week; the second because having settled down for a ten-minute chat the patient may then introduce the real reason for the consultation as he has his hand on the door, making his exit; the third over-runs because patients may recognise that if they want action on a problem he is the doctor to consult. His days are therefore full of decision-making — a time-consuming task.

Thus at the end of surgery each partner could claim to have worked a certain length of time, but the nature and value of the work done may have varied considerably. In calculating the number of appointments needed per session or per week, the partners must decide how effective each is in delivering their portion of primary care.

Like every other aspect of our work, we should look critically at our consulting speed. If we consistently get through patients at twelve to the hour, are we giving them enough time to talk? On the other hand, if we are taking ten or more minutes for each patient, is it because our consultation technique is too woolly and ineffective? These are difficult questions to answer, and most doctors will rationalise their behaviour. The speedy believe that patients with simple problems are dealt with very quickly, leaving enough time to be devoted to others who need more. The slow say that their patients are more satisfied, as they have had time to say all they want to. Very rarely have the doctors concerned tried to analyse what they are actually doing.

Recording consultations on tape or video is the only way to make some form of objective assessment of the process. There is now quite a lot of literature on the subject, with perhaps the most useful book being Byrne and Long, *Doctors Talking to Patients*. Listening to your own consultations should give you an insight into exactly what you are doing. You can then try and set objectives for improving technique and become confident that you are giving your patients what they need.

Although ideally partners should be seen to be doing equal 'work' by consulting at the same rate, some doctors may have to appreciate that they can only work effectively if they have more time than average per patient. In these cases a smaller surgery is fairer to the patients than a doctor who is continually trying to keep to time but inevitably running late.

Handling difficult people

Nothing can be as disturbing to the doctor's equilibrium as having to deal with a difficult patient or relative, especially in the middle of a busy surgery. Strategies have to be developed to handle these people, if not to their satisfaction, then certainly to everyone else's.

However, we should appreciate that the large majority of our patients are considerate and understanding and, if anything, do not stand up for themselves enough in their dealings with the medical profession. The aberrant behaviour of the few, while intensely annoying, should not be allowed to influence decisions about the level of service being provided to the practice as a whole.

Though the variety of difficult behaviours encountered may be great, there are some broad categories which can be considered.

1. Rejection of responsibility Most frequently, aberrant behaviour is the result of social, emotional or physical problems affecting the patient, and an understanding of this can make it easier to deal with some incidents. Some patients have neither the intellect nor the social skills to cope with situations which generate a lot of anxiety, particularly if this is associated with responsibility for the care of others.

Many young people manage to get to adult life and start a family without ever taking on much responsibility. When faced with difficulties which necessitate thoughtful action or decisions, they may react with panic or denial of responsibility. Anxiety coupled with the lack of maturity is perhaps the most frequent cause of difficulties. An example is the young parent who, when faced with a child with a cold, avoids making a decision about management by calling the doctor, so handing over the problem and the responsibility.

Rejection of responsibility as a cause of aggressive behaviour also occurs in other situations. Disaffected spouses, children who are resentful about having to look after parents, or neighbours who do not want to be involved with a sick person who is living alone are all examples of people who may make unreasonable demands. A classic case is the 'Sunday morning syndrome', where a son who is feeling guilty about not having paid enough attention to his parents visits them reluctantly and then calls out the doctor, demanding urgent treatment or admission.

Patients can of course be difficult without being rude or aggressive. We all allow ourselves to be used by manipulative people to a greater or lesser extent. They have learned to use social, emotional or physical problems to get what they want from the doctor. The need may be attention or drugs, or just a letter to the housing department. The most successful are those who make offers of illnesses that the doctor just cannot resist.

The strategy All doctors feel the need to be needed, and this is even more satisfying if we think that we are being therapeutically effective. The stroking of our self-image of being the potent healer makes us susceptible to the wiles of the patient who tells us how good we are, how we are needed and how no-one else will possibly do.

General practitioners on the whole find it difficult to manage manipulative patients. The doctor who is quite fierce with the overtly demanding patient may be like putty in the hands of the lady who gently strokes his ego while being far more demanding than any of the so-called difficult patients. A healthy cynicism about what one can or cannot do, or even about what it is appropriate to do for a patient, will help to avoid getting too emotionally involved. One should of course be kind and sympathetic, but at the same time firm. Patients have to be made to confront the fact that they are responsible for their own destinies and that consulting is not a way of making the doctor responsible for solving their emotional or social problems.

In any transaction with patients, it is important to identify who is responsible for what. Thus the patient who says that she wants to kill herself does not make you responsible for stopping her unless she is suffering from a clear-cut psychotic illness. In the same way, you are not responsible for solving social, emotional or interpersonal problems. You may offer help, but only as you see fit.

Being firm in this way does not stop the GP from taking a sympathetic interest in patients' problems, and very often defining roles improves the relationship. Once the rules of the transaction are established, it is easier to get down to work to help patients sort out their own problems and to develop insight.

The same principles of understanding, and appropriate sympathy coupled with unemotional firmness and education, can be used for coping with the other varieties of difficult patients.

Patients who are anxious because of immaturity and reluctance to take responsbility are less easy to handle at times. They and the patients who are demanding because they think that is the only way to get appropriate care must be shown that the practice is keen to give a good service. The principle is: agree first, argue and educate later. The father who rings up for a visit that is probably not necessary is best answered by: 'Yes, of course I shall come if it is necessary.' This defuses most aggression, because an offer of help has been made. You can then go on: 'But from what you are telling me it sounds as if it is just a feverish cold, and there is nothing very much that I shall be able to do.' If the father is still anxious for a visit, then go, but make sure that you reinforce your statement on the phone by not prescribing. This is the doctor's way of proving to the patient that the visit was not necessary.

Receptionists can work in the same way: 'Yes, of course we shall fit you in immediately if it is necessary — but the doctor is very busy, and if it is not an emergency, could it wait until — ?' If the patient insists on being seen and it is not necessary, then the education must be completed by the doctor not prescribing and giving information about what is or is not urgent.

2. *The impact of a serious illness* The impact of a serious illness may have profound effects on the behaviour of the patient or caring relatives. The woman who is mourning the loss of a breast or the tough docker who has just had a coronary may either get depressed and passive, or a build-up of tension may erupt in unexpected rudeness. An example is the normally compliant lady who had just had a mastectomy who came in and asked the receptionist for a certificate. When told that the doctor wanted to see her, she saw this as a rejection and told the waiting room at large what an uncaring lot they were in this practice.

The strategy Aggression caused by anxiety about some serious illness or problem is quite easy to handle, provided doctors and staff have the sensitivity not to take the behaviour at its face value. Very often you will have a good idea of the cause of the anxiety, and it is then important to confront the patient: 'You seem to be upset. You must be very worried about your recent operation on your breast.' This will usually lead to some emotional catharsis. Afterwards, explanation that the practice is always willing to help where possible and that there is no need for aggression can be given. Very often there is no need for the latter explanation, as the patient is very unlikely to be aggressive again after having been able to express pent-up feelings.

3. *'Psychopathic' personalities* A few patients have psychopathic personalities and will always act as if their own wishes or needs are of paramount importance. If they want any particular service, they will set about getting it in the way that they think will be most effective. If aggression appears to be the quickest way to get an appointment, then they will be aggressive, regardless of the effects on others. Alternatively, they may use dramatic but untruthful stories or sheer irresistible charm to get what they want.

The strategy These gratuitously aggressive patients are very difficult to educate. They need firm handling and should be told in no uncertain terms that, if they expect service and courtesy from the practice, they too will have to be polite and moderate their demands. A vigorous fight back by the doctor usually improves rather than damages relationships. Respect increases when the patient realises that the doctor is not to be browbeaten. If there is no evidence that an aggressor is sorry for his or her actions, then it is reasonable to consider removing the family from the list. This seems to be a very effective way of changing behaviour, as it is noticeable that patients who have been forced to leave become much less troublesome to their new doctor.

Before someone is thrown off the list, it is important to ask if you really think that the patient's behaviour will be altered by this action. If they are going to be just as bloody-minded with the next doctor, then it might be fairer if you held on to them and tried to develop some kind of relationship. You also have to ask yourself if your own or other practice members' behaviour was above reproach.

For some totally obnoxious patients, neighbouring doctors may have to come to some agreement about sharing their care on a rota system.

4. Iatrogenic aggression We also have to remember that patient behaviour is very much influenced by interaction with doctors and their staff. Aggression today might well be the result of past contacts thought by the patient to be unsatisfactory.

Where doctors have been very unwilling to visit or where it has been unreasonably difficult to get appointments, the patient may perceive the business of getting to see the doctor as a sort of war that has to be waged vigorously. Consequently, demands may be aggressive or the patient may elaborate stories to get quick results. The bad-tempered and uncommunicative doctor or the unfriendly, unskilled receptionist may generate these feelings in patients even when the service is quite good, if assessed objectively.

The strategy Doctors and staff members who consistently cause patients problems are unlikely to be perceptive enough either to fully appreciate what they are doing or to be honest enough to accept the responsibility for their actions and apologise.

Of course, this refers to doctors who work in isolation. Those in functional partnerships should have the effects of their behaviour drawn to their attention, with supportive discussion to help them to change. Staff with the same problem should also be supported and educated, though if this does not lead to the necessary improvements, then formal warnings and even dismissal may follow.

As far as the patient is concerned, the doctor who appreciates what has gone on should apologise sincerely, explain how the practice is meant to operate, and do perhaps a bit more than is necessary to ensure the patient leaves the surgery, if not completely satisfied, at least mollified.

Very few people are not disarmed by an honest admission of 'guilt' and an ungrudging apology. Many would find their anger increasing if it was met by a closing of ranks and a complete disbelief that any practice member could have acted in the way they have said. It takes a lot to make the average patient complain, and very often there may well be more than a grain of truth in the allegation.

Managing workload

Workload in practice is often discussed in rather emotive terms, and is usually assessed subjectively rather than objectively. It is very difficult to find out what people mean when they talk about their 'workload', though get any group of GPs together over a drink and, before the evening is out, you can be sure that the subject will rear its head in one guise or another.

Feelings on the subject are determined mainly by two factors: the amount of work actually being done and the perception of how useful, relevant and enjoyable it is. The doctor who sincerely believes that most of the work is relevant and appreciated by the patients will tolerate a higher case load than someone who is disenchanted and regards most of the problems as trivial.

The pace of work in general practice also colours attitudes. Some GPs complain about having to see patients at rates of one every five to ten minutes. One could easily get the impression that this goes on all day, but of course consulting actively is confined to only four hours or so. The pace of work at other times may well be quite lesiurely. Similarly, the amount of time partners spend away from the practice has a bearing on workload. For example, a practice of five taking six weeks' holiday and two weeks' study leave each per year is working with half a doctor less than if they were each only allowed four weeks off annually. Likewise, two half-day sessions and a whole day off adds up to only three-fifths of a doctor.

The total of hours worked per week varies enormously. The small group that does its own out-of-hours cover may chalk up an impressive total each week, while the doctors in another practice that gives each partner a full day off during the week and uses a deputising service may actually work only twenty or thirty hours a week. Naturally, the practitioner with a lot of time off may have to work quite intensively when actually in the surgery — but then, you cannot have your cake and eat it. The hours worked by British GPs are on the whole much less than those in other countries. This does not mean that the work is any less effective in medical terms.

Attempts at objective assessment of workload are almost as inaccurate as subjective ones. The common parameters used are the hours worked and consultation rates or items of service. These figures may give some idea about how long the worker is on the treadmill, but little information about how stressful or how effective it is. Seeing thirty patients in the surgery may sound like hard work, but if most of them are unnecessary repeats, quick certificates and simple colds, it may in fact be a very easy session. In these circumstances the problem cases that really need sorting out may be scared off by the sheer weight of numbers: 'I know how busy you are, doctor'. Another GP with only fifteen cases to see might be under considerable pressure if a lot of problem-solving is involved.

With all these variables it is very difficult to define what is a reasonable workload — and it must be reasonable, or else sooner or later the stress will tell. The chronically overworked doctor will become less enthusiastic about the job and performance will suffer.

Putting it in rather vague terms, we feel the GP should be busy enough to be stretched occasionally, while regularly doing enough to feel intellectually satisfied.

Of course, we are referring to practice workload. Self-inflicted injury in the form of overwhelming extrapractice commitments is totally within the control of the doctor or practice concerned. However much the extra money may be enjoyed, its gaining should not be at the expense of our first priority, namely practice patient care. If the candle is being burned at both ends, then it is unreasonable to run down the practice service to maintain other activities; it is far fairer either to take on another partner or shrink the other commitments to the time reasonably available for them.

Workload is often talked about as if it is an immutable fact of life, inflicted on long-suffering GPs by patients who are not open to persuasion. We would like to suggest that workload can be modified to a considerable degree. In any practice, changes can be made to both the quantity and the content of the demand. The doctor is also in a position to redistribute the work, delegating where necessary and stimulating demand where indicated.

MODIFYING PATIENT EXPECTATIONS

As we have already discussed in detail in an earlier chapter, patients can be educated to change both the quantity and the quality of their demands. The practice where doctors communicate with each other to the level of formulating common policies can teach patients appropriate self-management of common ailments. This takes time, patience and consistent behaviour from the doctors, and a lot of effort will be wasted if maverick partners prescribe inappropriately for the sake of a quick consultation.

In some areas with traditionally high workloads, neighbouring practices should discuss common problems and try to formulate a common policy. A small practice in an industrial town might find it difficult to stop inappropriate prescriptions and certificates if all the surrounding practices continued to hand them out. This could lead to professional and financial suicide. Cooperation and coordination would be needed, but one has to have a collection of doctors who would actually be willing to work in some harmony.

ALTERING DOCTOR BEHAVIOUR

Patient-initiated demand is often learned behaviour — expectations being shaped by the doctors.

Appreciating what's happening

General practitioners can easily generate a lot of extra work for themselves. If they are in single-handed practice, they just have to work harder to cope with the extra consultations, though their patients may suffer because the doctors always appear to be so busy. In a group practice, however, aberrant behaviour in one partner will throw a lot of work on to the others. Three common behaviours may be observed.

1. *The 'Aren't I the caring, careful doctor' syndrome* The rather insecure doctor who needs to be seen to be careful or who doubts his or her own judgments is likely to have a high recall or repeat visit rate. The level of anxiety in patients is likely to be raised if they have to be seen again and again for checks. Any illness will be regarded as serious if anxiety is detected in the doctor.

2. *The 'Repeat blood pressure' syndrome* Senior partners in particular are prone to fill up their surgeries with chronically ill people who attend ritually for some check-up that may be unnecessary, or at least does not need to be done so frequently. The characteristic patient is the little old lady who comes in every month, sits down and

proffers a bared arm for her blood pressure to be tested. In spite of the fact that her blood pressure has been normal for some years, the doctor has not been able to work up the courage to tell her that she now only needs to have it tested once or twice a year.

Large numbers of these unnecessary repeats clog up the appointment system, and this places an unfair burden on the other partners who have to deal with greater numbers of new patients.

The routine repeat is a nice, easy consultation. Take the blood pressure, have a quick chat, hand out a repeat prescription and then there is time for a little rest before the next patient arrives. New problems are much more stressful. If you want an easy life, get yourself a lot of 'chronic' patients and get them to come more often than they need to. Your appointment book will always be full, and you can then bask in the reputation of being a popular doctor while having the pleasure of doing relatively stress-free surgeries.

3. The 'I'm God' syndrome   The doctor who is unable to delegate believes that only he or she is competent enough to deal with all the clinical and administrative facets of practice; only a minimum of work is handed on to nurses, health visitors and other paramedical staff. Such doctors are also inclined to have the delusion that patients only like to consult a 'real doctor'. The discovery that some patients are more likely to confide in a sympathetic nurse can cause much ego-bruising.

Changing established behaviour

Established behaviour is difficult to change in anyone. So how do we set about trying to change behaviour in an individualistic, prickly and rather conceited group of people like general practitioners? As we have previously discussed, there are two main strategies:

1. Communication (see p. 85)   Regular meetings and discussions take place, in which partners are kind and supportive enough to each other to be able also to criticise. Problems and experiences are shared. With patients free to seek second opinions or to be seen by different doctors at any time, the practice can monitor what it is doing and quickly identify any partner whose behaviour in any situation is way out of line. Self-imposed mutual standards help prevent any individual falling into bizarre, bad or even dangerous habits of care.

2. Audit (see p. 241)   Certain patterns of behaviour are more easily audited than others. The 'Repeat blood pressure' syndrome can be easily recognised by looking at appointment bookings regularly. Any partner consistently booking up Mondays one, two, three or more weeks before the date is indulging him or herself and may take a hint if the topic is brought up in a roundabout, tactful way at a practice meeting.

The insecure doctor is fairly easily recognised, but difficult to do much about. Education, support and confidence-boosting measures can help, but the anxious doctor's anxiety is such that it drives him or her to check patients repeatedly, despite an understanding of what is happening.

For all of us, repeat consultations for specific conditions may be the result of habit or unthinking adherence to dogma. Occasional audit of what exactly one does in the surgery may indicate ways of cutting down on unnecessary work. For example, which, if any, cases of otitis media need to be asked to come back for re-examination of the ear? The prognosis for acute otitis media is good unless there has been a persistent discharge, a strong family history or a history of frequent attacks. The development of glue ear is certainly not a problem, as in the vast majority of children it is self-limiting. Would it then be reasonable only to follow up the children with risk factors and to tell other parents to bring their children back only if they develop a discharge or there is any suspicion of deafness? You may not agree with this, but at least you ought to examine all the evidence objectively rather than base behaviour on the premise that more care equates with better care, or on some ill-thought-out advice from an expert who in fact has no experience of primary care.

There are a large number of problems that need to be evaluated in this way, and every GP should be able to identify some unnecessary doctor-initiated work that could be eliminated without doing any harm to the patients.

DELEGATING DISPASSIONATELY

Delegation is another way in which significant changes can be made in patterns of work. Once again, emotions play a big part in policy decisions. GPs often have a possessive and rather restrictive view of their patients, and they may see any delegation of duties as an erosive influence on this relationship. What we really need to ask ourselves is whether this intense and exclusive relationship really benefits the doctor more than the patient.

One GP we know will not allow a nurse to do a simple job like syringing ears — 'I like to do it myself'. Yet he grumbles incessantly about his workload, and his long-suffering patients have to sit around for ages in the waiting room while he fiddles about, fulfilling his image of a personal doctor. Who gains? Surely he cannot be getting much satisfaction from carrying out this simple task, unless perhaps there is some deeper Freudian explanation for his predilection? The patient does not benefit — the service is less efficient and there is no evidence that there is any great psychological benefit to be derived from having one's ears syringed by the doctor.

In our own practice we have tried to note patients' reactions to delegation, and have found that in the vast majority of cases they accept this willingly, because they are interested in efficient care and not in maintaining an exclusive relationship with their doctor.

Some of the apprehension about delegation may also be rooted in long-standing fears about job security. By maintaining that only the doctor can carry out all the traditional functions of the general practitioner, we are creating a closed shop. Patients will always have to come to us for these services if no-one else can do the job.

If delegation is acceptable to the doctor and the patient (and we think that problems of acceptance lie with the doctors and not with the patients), then it makes good sense to encourage it. The doctor is freed from some routine tasks that do little to enhance the doctor–patient relationship, and the patient gets a more efficient service. Another important factor is the enhanced job satisfaction that is experienced by the ancillary staff who can cultivate new and interesting responsibilities.

We are convinced that appropriate delegation is to everybody's advantage. The whole range of our work should be looked at to determine who would perform what best. There is of course a limit to the fragmentation of care, and there may come a time when the patient is unable to determine who is in charge of the situation. A team approach is acceptable, provided that overall clinical control is seen to be in the hands of the GP and the patients have free access to him or her whenever they think fit. The patient must feel that the doctor has not handed over care and that he or she is always aware of what is going on.

Straightforward nursing procedures, immunisation and simple advice for minor illnesses is now commonly delegated to practice nurses or attached district nurses. This has almost become the norm in any efficient and progressive practice and seems to have been accepted enthusiastically by patients and staff. There is little doubt that these practices offer a better service to their patients, and this is appreciated. At its simplest level, there is no doubt that nurses apply a bandage better than most doctors.

To be realistic, delegation may generate extra work. Any service will be used, and you may have to take some care that you are not just dishing out free plasters for minor grazes. The total number of patients seen may rise, though the number seeing the doctor may fall appreciably. Delegation does not mean just shoving off the patient onto someone else. It does mean giving a better service by deploying resources to maximum effect.

A more controversial application of this principle is to train nurses to undertake tasks that are normally considered to be purely medical. A number of practices, including ours, have nurses who undertake the long-term surveillance of many chronic patients. Once hypertension or heart failure or diabetes has been stabilised, it is quite feasible for nurses to do many of the routine checks. They are just as capable of taking a blood pressure or checking the ankles for oedema or asking about breathlessness as we are. In fact, they are better at systematic checks than the average doctor, who gets more satisfaction from problem-solving.

Some initial assessment visits are also well within the capabilities of the well-trained nurse. Measles, chicken pox and sore throats are all conditions that are seen regularly by our nurses.

This level of delegation can only be undertaken if the training is appropriate. The doctor and the nurse must be quite satisfied that this is adequate, and the nurse should have the last word about whether any particular referral is appropriate. There must be good communications. It would be quite intolerable for the nurse if she did not feel that she could refer back to the doctor at any time. Support must be complete.

The doctor who has trained a support team capable of a wide range of duties can offer patients new services without suffering the stress of having to do everything personally. Sharing the load means more time for the patients, more effective control of chronic illnesses and more screening procedures. All this costs the practice very little, because 70 percent of the nurses' salaries are repaid by the FPC. The GP who is really interested in good medical care, rather than in cultivating the image of the omnipotent personal doctor, will find this very satisfying. Practising good medicine at a reasonable pace while looking after enough patients to maintain expertise is what we should all be aiming for.

From all this you will appreciate that our objective in modifying workload is not so much to reduce it as to redistribute it more effectively. In fact, the total amount of work done may well actually be greater, only it is done by different people for different purposes.

A regular feature of practice discussions should be the possibility of offering new services which are cost-effective. These should not be undertaken in fits of starry-eyed enthusiasm, but should be evaluated critically, using a yield-to-effort-involved ratio as the yardstick of likely practical value.

Maximising income

General practitioners should be business-minded. This means devoting time and energy to financial aspects of practice.

We are protected to a considerable extent from the hard realities of private enterprise by the repayment of rents; 70 percent reimbursement of the salaries of ancillary staff, and a significant expenses element in our own remuneration. Other expenses are, however, a direct debit on the practice income, though being eligible for tax relief means effectively operating with a 40–50 percent discount, and more.

A normal business spends money to provide services which will hopefully pay for themselves by attracting new customers. In general practice, however, investment of money in equipment or other facilities generates little or no direct return. Buy an ECG and you may feel satisfied that you are practising better medicine, though it is very unlikely that many patients will be so impressed by this that they will ask to change to your list. In general, patients select doctors mainly for historical, geographical or personal reasons. Unfortunately, the quality of the equipment and the level of health care being provided appears to play little part in the making of their choice.

We are therefore in a situation where practice expenses produce little or no direct return — apart from the, not to be underestimated, feeling of satisfaction that comes from providing a good service. As business-people we have to manage the practice in such a way that we produce sufficient profit to make us feel that we are being reasonably paid for our expertise and efforts. A good income increases job satisfaction and enthusiasm, so we need to maximise our profit while working within the constraints of a reasonable workload and the provision of a service which satisfies our conscience. Paradoxically, efficient high-earning practices may be the ones that also give patients a good service — particularly if much of their income is derived from preventative activity.

DECIDING SPENDING PRIORITIES

Expenses vary a lot from practice to practice. The major outgoings of rent and rates are repaid directly. Extras for equipment, decorations and furnishings are a relatively small proportion of the practice turnover, so it is surprising how parsimonious some GPs are. Is there really any excuse for peeling paint, tatty furniture and rusting equipment when the average annual turnover is about £30 000 to £40 000 per partner? The extra amount of money involved in making the surgery attractive, and providing the equipment compatible with modern standards, is not excessive, especially when one realises that it is all tax-deductible.

Another point to remember is that the gross remuneration of the profession takes into account the average level of expenses. If general practitioners spend more, then they will be paid more to make up for it. Unfortunately, some GPs spend very little themselves and just pocket the extra monies being reimbursed for the expenses incurred by more generous and forward-looking colleagues. As a group we should spend more, as it is in the long-term interests of both the doctors and the patients.

There is of course a limit to how much an individual can and should spend. A balance has to be drawn between the needs of the practice and the desire of the GP to enjoy a good income. Careful thought is needed before buying expensive equipment. It must be reasonably certain to improve the practice's effectiveness before being a worthwhile investment. A computer, a defibrillator or even an expensive ECG might give food for thought — the niggardly sums involved in purchasing nebulisers, peak flow meters, glucometers, speculae, scales and what have you barely need to be considered, certainly not by any established partnership — for example:

Four doctors buy an ECG machine for £800.
Purchase cost per doctor £200.
Ultimate cost per doctor £80–140 (after individual tax relief at top rate).

(NB: If everyone bought an ECG machine, the net cost would be nil, as the government would pay the money back in the expenses element of remuneration.)

It is also worth noting that comparison between high- and low-expense practices shows that the higher-spending practices invariably achieve a higher take-home pay per patient due to their better organisation and businesslike methods.

CULTIVATING BUSINESS SENSE

While the acquisitive instincts of some doctors would put a market trader to shame, others have such an unrealistic view of the world that business matters are accorded a very low priority. Partnerships can accommodate financial dreamers so long as at least one member is prepared to accept the responsibility for looking after the practice's financial affairs and organising everyone else to help. This is not the same as one partner dealing exclusively with the money without reference to the others or in such secrecy that someone might wonder what there is to hide. There must be absolute honesty and trust among partners, especially where money is concerned.

That said, every GP should appreciate that income is relatively fixed and is derived from the basic practice allowance and capitation fees. To increase yearly profits significantly, business efficiency has to be improved either to allow costs to be cut, more to be achieved for the same money or effort input, or income to be directly increased. This increase may be from enhanced fee for item-of-service payments or may be from the extrapractice sale of doctor time released by better organisation.

Remember, 70 percent of the wages of two full-time staff, or their equivalents, per GP are paid for by the FPC. This means that much work can be delegated at little cost to the doctor, and any practice which does not have its full complement of ancillary staff should find out why. In the same vein, activities carried out by health visitors, midwives, community nurses and so on are entirely funded by central government, regardless of how much they benefit GPs or their patients. Again, much work can be delegated or shared to allow improvements in standards of care, enhancement of everyone's job satisfaction and, possibly, an increase in income for the practice.

With any size of practice, organisation of labour helps smooth running, and staff and doctors have to be trained to claim routinely for everything that is legally allowable. By this we mean payments from the FPC and other organisations, but not payments from individual patients seeking services that fall outside our terms and conditions of service. Such private individual fees are very much discretionary and, while it is a good principle to charge up-to-date fees for those who can afford them, it is also both charitable and sensible to waive fees for those in straitened circumstances.

Doctors can never claim all that they are entitled to unless they are fully aware of all the regulations apertaining to fees and reimbursements. Read and reread the Red Book, even if you think that you are pretty sharp with all your claims. Are you getting every allowance that is due to you? Are you making a profit on injections given, by issuing FP10s for them and then claiming the cost back, plus a dispensing fee? Are you claiming the cost of any diagnostic agent, e.g. allergy testing solutions? Read the small print and, if you are in any doubt about anything, speak to the FPC finance officer. Generally they are very helpful individuals who try to make sure that GPs get any monies due to them.

Another source of useful financial information is provided by the weekly medical papers. *Medeconomics* in particular merits careful monthly perusal, though the problem-answering services of *Doctor* and *Pulse* can both provide top-class, free advice to anyone who cares to write to them.

OPTIMISING NHS FEES

A well-organised practice can considerably enhance its income by making the most of its opportunities to generate fee for item-of-service payments. Happily, most of these money-making activities directly improve the service to patients. While money should not decide clinical practice, where good standards can attract extra income then that income can be justly viewed as both an incentive and a reward.

Areas to consider

1. Immunisation (see p. 223)   With a bit of organisation, this can be quite a moneyspinner. The most important group are of course the children (see p. 223), and every practice should have a planned approach to this aspect of their care. One child having all vaccinations (up to preschool booster) from the practice will bring in £24.80 in fees, and an 80 percent uptake rate among the 30 babies on an average GP's list will yield £595.20 per GP per year.

Overseas travellers (see p. 22) also benefit from immunisations and advice. The requirements for individual countries can be complex, so one partner should be given the job of keeping up to date with developments. Again, a systematic approach allows doctor involvement to be minimal (about 2–3 minutes at the most for the average patient), with receptionists and nurses carrying out the real work. An overseas traveller going to an underdeveloped country will bring in at least £22.30 in fees and charges — a sum worthy of a little effort.

A few hours spent organising and training can save doctors work, directly and from the decrease in infectious diseases among patients, earn extra money and provide a better service.

Though an aggressive immunisation policy is good medicine and good busines, it should still be critically assessed from time to time. Only those procedures that are genuinely going to benefit patients should be performed. Rubella screening and vaccination is so medically effective that it should be performed despite the likely poor return, if assessed in purely financial terms.

Devising methods of keeping everyone's tetanus immunisations up to date (a booster is necessary medically every ten years, not the every five years that the FPC will pay for) is both medically and financially sensible.

Influenza vaccination for at-risk groups, on the other hand, should probably not be done, despite the guaranteed extra income it might offer, as it could be argued the medical value is uncertain.

2. *Contraception* Again a confident, aggressive approach by the whole practice can sell a worthwhile service to the public. High practice standards can retain patient loyalty and so maintain a regular income while improving contraceptive efficacy.

Well-motivated family planning trained GPs can provide a service to even the most poorly motivated of their patients. Twenty percent of patients are females in their reproductive years, and it is likely that most, at some time, will require or would benefit from contraceptive advice. As they consult on average five times each a year, there are many opportunities to discuss and review their contraceptive needs. The GP is in an excellent position both to give advice and to implant attitudes and practices that may benefit the patient and her family for years to come.

Ideally, the notes of every patient of reproductive potential should contain a clear record of their current need for or method of contraception. This enables the doctor to identify these patients, who can be asked tactfully about their contraceptive needs and perhaps be made aware of other options that may be open to them. Some situations, e.g. patients new to the practice, women with genitourinary symptoms, young women consulting with apparently minor problems, are more 'fertile' ground for this sort of enquiry than others. However, so long as the doctor is sensitive and obviously concerned with helping the patient, no offence is likely to be given or taken.

Having ascertained what is going on, it is important to keep a sense of proportion in deciding what to do with the information. Couples realistically and happily using methods such as the sheath or even coitus interruptus should be left well alone or, at the most, given advice as to how their chosen method might be more efficiently applied, or offered the prospect of alternative advice should they desire it in the future.

GP family planning services are freely available to all female patients; males are excluded. FP 1001s and 1002s have to be signed by both patient and doctor, and cover contraceptive services for twelve months from the date of acceptance. GPs may provide contraceptive services to patients not registered with them for general medical services. Also women are entitled to seek contraceptive advice from their GP and from a clinic at the same time. Attendance at a family planning clinic in itself does not preclude the general practitioner from giving contraceptive advice or treatment or from claiming for payment. This does not mean there is a free season on 'poaching' of patients who are happily attending a clinic and do not want advice from their GP.

Contraceptive care is well paid and a GP with the average 100 patients registered for contraception will earn £855 p.a.

3. *Smear-taking* This is another worthwhile activity which should be undertaken for its medical effectiveness and not for the income it may generate. Certainly fifth-yearly smears in the over-35s, or women who have had three pregnancies, will attract a fee, but it does not compensate for the work involved. Also, there is no fee payable for the women, under 35, particularly with multiple sexual partners or early first intercourse, who now seem to be increasingly at risk of developing carcinoma *in situ*.

An intrapractice smear clinic run by the practice nurse can generate enough income to pay part of the costs. The rest of the cost must be borne by the practice, though even if no smears attracted a fee, the practice should still provide this service.

4. *Antenatal care* On average, each GP will have 30 antenatal patients to claim for in a 'year'. Overall, in 80 percent of cases care is shared with consultants and in only 20 percent does the GP take complete responsibility, including being responsible for the care

given by the midwife during labour. In less than 1 percent of cases will a GP actually be involved in labour care. For the provision of antenatal and postnatal care, a GP on the obstetric list will earn about £2266 p.a. — with an additional £20 or so per patient under full care.

The prospect of increasing work to increase income is limited to only two areas. One is by taking full responsibility for care in as many cases as it is clinically correct to do so, and the other is to carry out the maximum reimbursable postnatal visits allowable, namely five, in shared-care patients discharged from hospital after 48 hours. Each GP/practice has to decide whether the £20 or so in the first instance or the £3.00 per visit in the second represents a decent return for the likely time/expense involved and whether the likely patient satisfaction engendered would outweigh the value of other activities that the doctor could be indulging in. We do not believe that 5 postnatal visits are medically necessary. Our policy is to do only one routine postnatal visit unless the patient has been discharged in less than 48 hours when we would do two.

Most of the points to consider carefully to maximise the benefits to all concerned are covered on p. 60 and p. 238. The only additional one we would like to make is that only partners on the obstetrics list should look after maternity cases. Not only do they attract far higher fees, but there is evidence that the care they give may be better for the patients.

Claiming religiously

One problem of an item-of-service system is that the practice has to be methodical about claiming. In each practice one or two of the staff should be responsible for the claims, though everybody must know about the system. If too many people get involved, there may be confusion. A system should be established for checking each type of form and this should be adhered to rigidly, otherwise some claims will be missed. However, do not get too carried away in your efforts to glean every last penny. If the administration is too complicated, the staff will never operate efficiently, so any system has to be cost-effective. Complicated systems or computers are expensive in time and money and have to demonstrate that they will save enough money to make their use worthwhile.

A common reason for lost fees is missing claim forms for immunisations. They should be filled in and sent off to the FPC after each immunisation is done and not retained until a course is finished. This may not be too popular with the FPC, but you are entitled to do this and it saves a lot of bother. Some patients never complete their courses of injections, and just having the forms around for three months or so invites problems.

Maternity claim forms are another potential source of lost revenue. The book in which the forms arrive may be used to record when they should be sent off. If you want an additional safeguard, the notes of each antenatal patient can be extracted and filed separately. They are also further identified with a label being stapled onto the front of the envelope. When the pregnancy is over and the postnatal is done, the record is not returned to the file until the label is removed and the claim form completed.

Family planning claims have the additional complication that they have to be renewed each year. It is easy to forget when the next claim is due, and it is no use relying on the patient bringing along her slip of paper with the details of the last claim. The easiest method is to write FP 1001 or 1002 in red on the notes, on the date of the original claim and preferably on a custom-designed contraception card. If this can be easily identified, then subsequent claims should not be forgotten. A back-up system is to file the doctor's section of the form under the month when the renewal is due. This can act as a reminder and can also be used to chase up defaulters. This particularly applies to patients on the coil or the cap who should come in for an annual check, but forget. Pill patients are easier, because they have to come back to get their supply of the tablets.

Informing patients of practice services

While advertising by doctors is strictly forbidden, intrapractice advertising or 'informing patients of the services being provided' is a perfectly respectable activity. Of course, the kind of notice used in one-practice premises may well be very different from that allowed or prudent for a multipractice health centre where other practices' patients may be influenced. No-one can object to a doctor informing his or her patients only, though if any difficulties or doubts are experienced, a phone call to the FPC, LMC or BMA should provide the correct procedure.

If you give a first-class contraceptive service, patients soon get to know about this and more of them are likely to approach you for advice. You can also discreetly advertise the fact that the practice likes to be involved in contraception. Many patients assume that the general practitioner is not really interested, and they may go to a local authority clinic because they do not want to add to their doctor's workload.

This is one argument for having a practice information leaflet that can be given to all new patients. Copies can also be left in the waiting room for anybody to pick up. All the practice services can be advertised in this way, and it can also be used to give information about surgery times, requests for visits, etc. A small notice in the waiting room may also help.

Contraception is the province of the general practitioner and, even if we were not paid for it, we should be making a specific effort to encourage our patients to use the service. The fact that we can make a considerable amount of money in this way is incidental, though we should be businesslike enough to make the most of the opportunity.

Notices should also draw patients' attention to the times that immunisations will be available, the need for medical advice before an overseas journey, the need for and availability of the practice cytology service, and so on. Information presented in this way can jog the patient's memory and increase trade!

DISCERNING PRIVATE INCOME

Fees from the FPC are not the only source of income open to practices. There are all manner of jobs, both in or out of the NHS, which can produce reasonable supplements to income. Any extra commitments, however, will affect the practice's ability to give an optimal service to patients. The extra income and extra interest provided by another job must be carefully balanced against the difficulties of doing justice to partners, practice and the new post. All partners should agree before one is allowed to accept any new work, and ideally the income should go into the pool.

Industrial clinics, children's clinics, family planning clinics are all suitable part-time work for general practitioners. If possible, they should be timed so that they do not interfere with normal surgeries. Clinical assistantships in local hospitals allow the pursuit of special interests, but anyone doing them should be careful not to be lumbered with a dull job that no-one else wants.

The clinical assistant in hospital should be in a job in which there will be an educational as well as a service commitment. The average haematology session consists of managing the anticoagulant clinic, whilst the surgical assistant merely injects varicose veins all afternoon. Both jobs have limited value. Far better to choose a dermatology or rheumatology job for about a year, liaise with and learn from an enthusiastic consultant, and then both the GP and practice patients will benefit in the future.

Training and teaching provides another source of income. A trainer's allowance is now quite a lucrative addition, especially as a trainee in the practice should also do a reasonable amount of work to gain enough experience. These are not easy pickings, however, as the requirements for training practices are getting ever more stringent. A substantial amount of time must be devoted to the trainee, and the practice itself must be well organised. A trainer will not be expected to have much in the way of other work commitments, so there will be restrictions on the ability to earn money from other sources.

A course organiser gets the same reward as a trainer, but the work involved is such that it is not an economically viable post. You do it because you enjoy it, not for the money. The same might be said about trainers, especially in group practices where the divided, taxed income leaves little tangible reward for all the time and effort.

RENDERING UNTO CAESAR

Honesty in the practice we have already touched on. All the partners should have access to the accounts at all times. As with everything else, frequent discussions will avoid misunderstandings about financial matters. Regular reviews avoid having too much money lying around in the bank or the development of an embarrassing overdraft.

Honesty with others is equally important. The relationship with the taxman in particular is less stressful when there really is nothing to be concealed. Tax evasion is unlawful and, for a professional person like a GP, carries the additional penalty of public opprobrium should discovery be publicised. Tax avoidance is a different kettle of fish, and the struggle to keep as much of one's money as is legally possible is both stimulating and rewarding.

While *Money which?* tax guides and the financial columns of daily and medical papers give much good advice, the key to success is a good accountant who will not only help the practice but will help individual GPs to help themselves. The best accountants are likely to handle the affairs of several GPs and therefore are acquainted with the peculiar financial problems and tax allowances to which we are entitled.

Of course, the accountant needs help. The practice financial whizzkid should keep full accounts (or have someone regularly keep them in his or her stead) to present. This not only makes the accountant's job easier; it also makes sure that nothing is forgotten, thus gaining the partners their full entitlements and cutting the accounting bill. Individual doctors should work on the same principles.

Get into the habit of keeping an account of any money spent on articles (including petrol and other motoring expenses) connected in any way with the conduct of practice business. Although we cannot even begin to cover what can be claimed, remember the little details like film for the camera if you take any clinical photographs. These all mount up over the years.

Also you can buy good pictures or furniture for the surgery. Their value will be written down (depreciated) year by year in the accounts until the practice ends up with some nice articles which, despite having no further accounting value, have their intrinsic value and are a pleasure to own.

Remaining friendly with colleagues

General practice is gradually emerging from the traditional isolationism that has been engendered by the competitive nature of the business. In the past, normal behaviour comprised observing the ethical rules and being polite to each other while avoiding contact for the purpose of mutual education or the formulation of policies. The code of ethics gave some structure to relationships, but there was little in the way of warmth or mutual support.

As the NHS became established and competitiveness decreased, at least in some areas, GPs began to realise that they could help each other. At its simplest level, this cooperation took the form of rotas for out-of-hours duties, and for the first time it became accepted for general practitioners to get together to discuss problems of practice organisation. They also took the unprecedented step of allowing rivals to see their patients.

At a more sophisticated level, general practitioners began to realise that they could teach and learn from each other, and exploratory groups or 'workshops' were set up. Balint groups and the emerging College were other forces encouraging greater contact among enquiring minds.

FOSTERING GOOD INTERPRACTICE RELATIONSHIPS

The two factors which enhance relationships with neighbouring practices are good communications and strict adherence to accepted ethical standards. The BMA has an established code of ethics which should be studied by everybody, members or not. The most important rules affecting relationships with colleagues are those concerning advertising and not seeing each other's patients without permission.

Unfortunately, there is some evidence that these codes are not being as strictly observed as they should be. Advertising or the canvassing of patients can never be condoned. No matter how difficult the problems, one should never be tempted into trying to attract patients in this way. Not only is it unethical and likely to make the perpetrator an outcast among local colleagues, but it is plainly counter-productive. Patients are generally quite astute, and they are well aware that doctors are not supposed to indulge in these activities. If they are canvassed, they are more than likely to take offence, and the offending doctor's reputation will be demeaned in the locality.

Working in an off-duty rota, it is inevitable that you will have to see the patients of colleagues. This calls for some tact and sensitivity. Sometimes a particular management regime will appear to be inappropriate, but the temptation to change treatment must be resisted unless there is some emergency. Direct or even implied criticism must be avoided at all costs, as it will only engender resentment and retaliation. For the same reasons, it is wise not to take someone on to the list who has been seen while you are deputising.

Another source of friction is seeing patients without the permission or knowledge of their regular GP. For some reason, doctors appear to believe that the normal ethical standards only apply to NHS patients and that, if a patient asks to be seen privately, the usual courtesies are unnecessary. If we are ever in this position, we always ring up the patient's GP and ask for permission and for any medical details we ought to know. Not only is this ethical, but it is also prudent. Such patients are often in the process of manipulating their medical advisers, and you can find yourself in some difficulties if you do not know exactly what has been going on. It is also worth considering that a patient may be taking drugs that you are not aware of. This could be dangerous for the patient as well as being risky from the medico-legal point of view.

The best insurance against bad feelings among colleagues is to make sure that there is a reasonable amount of social and academic contact among different practices. A local medical club or a local branch of the Ladies Medical Guild can organise dinners, dances and similar events. When doctors can meet and talk things over, resentments and misunderstandings are less likely to arise. Involvement in local medical politics can be another good way of making contact with fellow GPs.

TREATING HOSPITAL DOCTORS AS ALLIES

Relationships with consultants are governed by the same principles of good ethics, good practice and good communications. Hospital colleagues can be met at local postgraduate centres, particularly at lunch and meetings. As with GP colleagues, social chat can be a great preventer or healer of misunderstandings.

High standards of practice and appropriate use of the specialist services will earn the respect of hospital colleagues. Your ego is not the only beneficiary, as your patients will also be helped, since any request from you for an urgent appointment or other action will be taken more seriously.

If GPs expect to be allowed to speak to consultants on the phone when they think fit, then they too should be willing to be available whenever hospital staff try to contact them. Many consultants become infuriated by the protective behaviour of practice staff (perhaps forgetting how difficult it can be for GPs to contact them). However, it is reasonable to make sure that reception staff know exactly who can be put straight through on the phone or given your ex-directory telephone number to allow contact at home.

Junior hospital staff should be treated with exactly the same courtesy as their more senior colleagues. This can pay off handsomely when trying to get a geriatric patient into hospital in the middle of the night.

RESPECTING EVERYONE ELSE!

Doctors are not the only professional colleagues with whom GPs have to work. It is just as important to establish happy relationships with health visitors, district nurses and social workers as with other GPs — perhaps even more so. Though it may be anathema to some doctors, it certainly improvees relationships if nurses, chemists, social workers and so on are treated by practice staff in the same way as other doctors would be. This means with respect and a high priority for action.

Patients are best served if the group of professionals involved in their care actually talk to each other, even to the extent of agreeing about what management would be best in a particular situation. This relationship cannot succeed unless paramedicals are treated with respect and viewed as colleagues rather than as servants to the omnipotent doctor. Once again, meetings are essential, and the practice timetable must be organised so that regular discussions can take place.

A considerable amount of tact and understanding is needed to cope with the attitudes of some of these colleagues. Health visitors, nurses and social workers are all in the process of redefining their professional roles, and sometimes they are particularly sensitive about their status. This may on occasion lead to them striking what may appear to be rather aggressive postures. This is symptomatic of their insecurity, and the GP may have to be careful not to give the impression of trying to exercise direct control. To be realistic, there will be times when the doctor has to take control of the situation, but this can be done tactfully, and 'advice' will invariably be accepted in a crisis, if only because it is well recognised that the ultimate responsibility in most cases does lie with the doctor.

Once again, the social meeting can work wonders for relationships, and the occasional meeting over a drink and sandwiches is well worthwile.

Remembering your family and yourself

So far, we have talked at some length about the need for GPs to give a good service, and how keeping up to date and indulging in other academic activities helps to improve standards of practice. This implies a willingness to work hard, though employing strategies such as delegation and patient education may modify the load to tolerable levels. Our philosophy does not imply a total and exclusive commitment to general practice, nor should work be used as an escape from social and emotional problems.

Workaholism is a well recognised syndrome, and one of the prominent symptoms is marital pathology. There are a few extraordinary people who manage an astonishing amount of academic or political work and still manage to stay friends with their spouses and partners. One can only admire their abilities, but one suspects that the qualities of the spouses and partners may be the more important in maintaining this happy situation. We ordinary mortals must take care to look after the needs of our families — not to mention ourselves.

SPOUSES AND CHILDREN FIRST

Because of changing attitudes towards surgery hours and the common use of appointment systems, the working hours of general practitioners are now quite flexible. Gone are the days when every GP, simply because competing GPs were doing the same, did an evening surgery which did not end until eight or nine at night. This often meant that the kids were in bed by the time Dad got home, and if they were at school he did not see them in the afternoons either. Daddy was just the strange man who appeared at weekends (at least we hope it was Daddy!).

Make sure you are at home enough actually to have some fun with the children. Do not forget that your spouse also needs to see you and may not want to share you with the children all the time. Having some sort of regular relaxation helps everyone. For some this means socialising, while for others it may mean digging in the garden or sailing. If you become involved in a vicious circle of frenetic activity, you may suddenly find that you no longer have time for relaxing, and this in the long run is likely to make you function less efficiently.

Every now and then take stock of what you are doing and ask yourself if the balance of activity is right. Sometimes a series of new commitments makes it difficult to find spare time. If this is unavoidable for a while, it is reasonable to carry on, provided you have a clear plan for the not too distant future which will allow you and your family to resume a balanced life.

One way in which a practice can ensure at least a minimum of social activity is to organise regular practice outings. This does not mean that the partners' families should live in each other's pockets, but it does give spouses an opportunity to meet each other and the other partners socially. It is also a way of saying thank you for all the times wives or husbands have had to stay at home while the partners have been out at meetings or other practice business. Similarly, if you belong to committees or faculty boards, which entail going to evening meetings, then try and persuade colleagues in that organisation to have at least one or two social events a year.

ALL WORK AND NO PLAY

It is of course important to get away from things medical and from medical people. There is too much to do and enjoy in life to restrict interests to the narrow and sometimes claustrophobic world of medicine. If for no other reason, remember that one day retirement will loom and nothing could be worse than to discover that work has left no time for any other interests or activities.

The nature of outside interests matters not a bit, though one has to be reasonable — it may just put partners out a bit if one of their number was a well-publicised spokesman for the gay liberation front or was regularly up before the beaks for kicking policemen's horses on ban-the-bomb demonstrations. Hobbies in our practice vary from playing the violin, to keeping bees, to breeding rare species of frogs. Mind you — some of these hobbies can themselves cause family disruption, but that is another story.

REGISTERING WITH A GP

Doctors are very bad at being patients and are likely to be less than perfect when it comes to managing the medical care of their own families. In many practices the families are registered with the other partners though most if not all the day-to-day medical care is handed out by the parent or spouse who is the doctor.

There is a good argument for partners and their families being registered with another practice. In many situations there may be a conflict of interests, particularly with long-term physical illness, any psychiatric illness or with social and emotional problems. These may all profoundly affect the running of the practice, and a partner's professional detachment is bound to be modified by other considerations. In these situations it would be much better to have an independent practitioner, possibly a consultant colleague (though some risk of over-investigation and over-treatment would have to be run) who could give objective advice.

Undertaking the medical care of ourselves and our families is full of pitfalls. As a group we tend to fall into one of two categories — the alarmists and the excessively sanguine. The alarmists see sinister reasons for every symptom. Every sore throat will get belted with penicillin (or whichever sample of an antibiotic just happens to be lying about). The sanguine can never believe that it could happen to them. They will complain about the wife's nerves as she goes obviously thyrotoxic, or suck Rennies for indigestion as they are in the throes of their first coronary.

If in doubt, get some senisble and independent advice. Ask for it as a patient and not as a colleague. You will make things very difficult for the unfortunate person you consult if you do not take on the patient's role in this transaction. It would be most unfair to start off by saying, 'Do you think this pain in my back could be due to playing too much golf last week?' The doctor would not know whether to make a fairly casual comment on your suggestion or a real diagnostic effort. Instead of suggesting the diagnosis, which is very difficult to ignore, coming from a colleague, it would be much better to offer the symptom in a manner which would allow the person you consulted to follow any diagnostic pathway he or she wished.

Your family should be encouraged to seek help from other doctors, and you should not be put out if they bypass you. Remember that they may have problems or worries that they do not want you to know about. This particularly applies to your children as they get into their teens and want to be more independent.

Take care of yourself and the family at least as well as of your patients. Have you or your spouse had a blood pressure check in the last five years? Are your tetanus and other immunisations up to date? It would be quite likely that in a practice busily engaged in screening for hypertension that the partners would forget to include each other in the process.

Section 4
Keeping the team harmonious

Introduction

Today's general practitioner does not work in isolation. The financial power to employ staff, the trend towards group practice and the willingness of health authorities to attach staff has led more and more to the sharing and delegation of work.

Virtually every practice now has some help from secretaries and receptionists. At least 80 percent also have one or more nurses working with them, either on attachment from the DHA or as direct employees. However, even amongst practices that have their full quotas of staff and attachments, many have failed to make the best use of the range of talent so readily available to them.

Above all else, successful teamwork is dependent on the fostering of a strong belief among all the participants that they are essential members of the practice, responsible for working together to provide the highest possible standard of primary care.

The team is dead, long live the team

Some fifty or so years ago, before the Second World War, it became increasingly apparent that general practitioners and private nurses could not and would not be able to provide all the primary medical care needed by the population. To fill the huge gaps in care that existed, local authorities were empowered to provide home nursing and midwifery and free medical supervision for expectant mothers and children. Infant mortality was still appallingly high and, to improve standards of child care, a new role was created for specialised nurses who evolved into the health visitors of today.

So, when the NHS started, primary care was being provided by a variety of professionals, with separate though overlapping jobs. However, GPs were allowed to retain their independent and self-employed status, while the others continued to be employed by local authorities. The inception of the NHS therefore did little to integrate the functions of these workers and hardly helped the development of comprehensive primary care.

Over the past twenty to thirty years, the increasing awareness of the need for ancillary help in the surgery has been paralleled by a growing realisation that patients' needs can be met more appropriately and efficiently if nurses, health visitors, midwives and doctors work more closely together.

In 1958 the first experimental attachments of health visitors and district nurses took place. These early attachments were very successful, probably because they involved enthusiasts who were already sold on the idea. The early successes and the resulting propaganda led to the widespread adoption of the practice, and within a relatively short space of time many authorities redeployed their nurses and health visitors onto an attached rather than a geographical basis.

This blanket application of attachment schemes led to some disillusionment. Many GPs and nurses were not well motivated to work together, and cooperation was hampered by mutual scorn and mistrust. This was partly due to the lack of recognition by some GPs that nurses and health visitors had been busy upgrading their professional status and so were less inclined to regard themselves as hand maidens to the medical profession. These feelings, handled insensitively by GPs who saw themselves as automatic directors of the team, led to a lot of antagonism. The problems were then compounded by personality clashes and poor communications, which served to reinforce prejudices. In some areas the results have been so poor that the authorities have begun to redeploy their staff again — this time back onto a geographical basis.

Despite these setbacks, the concept of patient care by a team has gained increasing acceptance among general practitioners. Indeed, so uncritical has this acceptance been in some quarters that one cannot but wonder whether the main attraction has been the potential for reducing work by delegation rather than the potential for increasing the appropriateness and the effectiveness of patient care. While the former is a perfectly valid goal, it should not be pursued at the expense of the latter.

A SACRED COW?

The 'primary health care team' has now been elevated to the status of a sacred cow and rests on a vast mound of literature, extolling the virtues of cooperation between disciplines and the integration of care. Objective evidence for the effectiveness of teamwork, however, is hard to find, and little attention has been paid to the difficulties of coping with the realities of everyday practice. The 'team' has now become all things to all men, and one writer's picture may be that of an equal-status commune, while another's is that of a subservient team led by a whip-cracking doctor.

In truth, the word 'team' may not always be the most appropriate term for this diverse collection of people. Employed by different agencies; with a background of independent learning requirements; with a wide range of skills, abilities and responsibilities; and often working independently of each other with only peripheral coordination of their tasks, it is easy to see how they often do not function as an integrated team. In some instances there is no team approach of any sort, and network care is being provided (Table 4.1).

Table 4.1

Team care	Network care
Is provided by a small, clearly bonded group unchanging in identity over a long period of time in face-to-face work, often together, sharing values and outlook. Has a definite institutional base. Will always have some issue of leadership.	Is provided by interaction between a range of professionals who may not know each other personally and who do not have to consider each other's acceptability. No permanent or definite face-to-face group activity exists and individuals may come and go according to duty systems, shifts and rotas.

As the primary care 'team' can be so disparate, it is perhaps helpful to think of each member as a musician responsible for playing a different instrument. Although all should be professionally competent, it may be quite difficult to get them to play in harmony. Individual members must be willing to cooperate so that their own performance is of as high a standard as possible while, at the same time, their skills are used to strengthen the combined effect of the entire orchestra. The whole group must rehearse together and avoid the disharmony that comes from personality clashes, lack of individual motivation and inability to evolve some sort of leadership structure.

Many primary health care teams work superbly. Well-motivated people, willing to trust each other and to discuss problems, work together efficiently to evolve new and better standards of care. Sadly, as many teams are teams in name only with individuals who have not been mutually selected, but thrown together by chance and the whims of administrators. Not uncommonly, this leads to personal and ideological clashes which may be accentuated by professional jealousies engendered by the attitudes of the controlling hierarchies. Unfortunately, senior members of the various professions are too often obsessed by their own petty bureaucracies and status, and so fail to grasp the opportunities for advancing the roles of their colleagues who work in primary care.

Leading the pack

To function adequately, any group needs some form of leadership. This does not have to be obtrusive or directive, as subtle encouragement and benevolent manipulation is usually far more effective. Any member or members of a group may take on the role of leader though, to be realistic, the responsibility generally ends up with the practitioners concerned and, if they do not take on the job, it will go by default. Occasionally, a bright and personable nurse or health visitor will take the situation in hand and quietly manipulate all the others.

Given the present state of the health services, GPs who wish to maximise the effectiveness of their practices and to experiment with new methods of care have to make a realistic assessment of the nature of the team that is actually available for them to work with. Then a gradual process to modify attitudes and methods of work can begin and can achieve its aims with diplomacy, education and suitably subtle leadership. Where the group members are employed by the DHA and are controlled by their own hierarchies, change is much more difficult to achieve, and one has to keep a dialogue going, no matter how irritating the circumstances. Patience and diplomacy are often rewarded by surprising changes in attitudes, which make the effort worthwhile.

Staff employed by GPs are more easily influenced, both because they will have been personally selected and because 'he who pays the piper calls the tune'. However, even here leadership should be by discussion and education, as didactic direction can be counterproductive. The advantages of employing staff who can identify wholly with the needs and aims of the practice are so great that some GPs are employing not only nurses but also other professionals directly. Some trail-blazing practices now have their own health visitors, midwives and social workers. The reported success of some of these experiments and our own experiences lead us to believe that a full range of practice-employed staff offers progressive practices far greater prospects for flexible and rapid advancement than any amount of cooperation with Salmonised superstructures.

THE VALUE OF TEAMWORK

There are many advantages to teamwork. An obvious one is the economy gained by sharing facilities such as accommodation and support staff. The economies of scale also allow larger groups to utilise more sophisticated and expensive equipment. More importantly, however, it allows tasks to be performed by those who have the appropriate skills and time for them.

Team members, like health visitors and district nurses, bring with them special skills and attitudes which enable them to give some patients more appropriate care — it may be difficult to define precisely which patients. The routine surveillance of children and feeding problems might well be regarded as appropriate work for the health visitor, and the treatment of varicose ulcers the province of the district nurse, yet any of these jobs might be done by the general practitioner. Who actually does what in a particular situation will depend on the whims of the patient, doctor or nurse.

With team care, the patient has more appropriate access to a wider range of skills with, often, more time spent on the problem. For the team members there is the opportunity to delegate work to each other, ensuring that the best person deals with each particular patient.

A neglected and somewhat undervalued aspect of teamwork is the pleasure and intellectual stimulation of working with other people. There can be a continuous process of mutual education, with the pooling of ideas and knowledge, which can provide an immensely stimulating working environment. New policies and strategies can be developed, and patients will eventually benefit through the introduction of better systems of care.

To gain the maximum advantage from teamwork, a conscious effort is needed to maintain a high level of communication among all the members of the team. Even the simple expedient of arranging timetables so that people are free and together at certain times in the week will do much to make sure that they actually talk to each other.

THE HAZARDS OF TEAMWORK

A major disadvantage of teamwork is the very real possibility of personality clashes. They can lead to the breakdown of communications and to the provision of a disjointed service to patients. This is particularly likely to occur with attached rather than employed staff. However, it is not at all unusual for partners to fall out, a state of affairs which hardly sets a good example to the rest of the team. It is particularly important therefore for the doctors to put their own house in order and to develop common attitudes and policies before expecting the rest of the team to work together efficiently.

Another potential hazard of team care is that of allowing responsibility to become diluted. When the care of a patient is already shared with partners, further delegation to other team members can make it quite difficult to determine exactly who is responsible for the patient at any given time. Once again, the bigger the team, the more important it is to guard against this happening. To some extent good communications will make this hazard less likely, but it is important to make definite decisions about who is responsible for what.

Finally, with no control over selection, some practices will find that the quality of their attached staff leaves a lot to be desired. This presents enormous difficulties, and the only possible remedy is the use of friendly but persistent attempts at re-education.

Effective teamwork is undoubtedly a consumer of time. In a busy practice this may be in short supply but, unless time is set aside for the business of regular meetings and discussions, the team will never become a truly integrated and synergistic group.

Employing responsibly

The general practitioner employer has certain responsibilities, both legal and moral. Employed staff have much the same needs as the doctors themselves. Good pay, good conditions of work and happy relationships are essential if people are to give of their best. Job satisfaction, intellectual stimulation and a feeling that their views and ideas will always be taken seriously helps to keep staff interested in and loyal to the practice.

Many practices have underpaid their staff for years and have taken advantage of the fact that many people consider it a privilege to work in a doctor's surgery. This is an indefensible attitude, and GPs must take care to pay their staff properly. The appropriate Whitley council rates, which are paid to health authority employees doing the same jobs, give a good guide to the minimum acceptable levels.

It is difficult to understand the meanness of some practices when 70 percent of the wages are reimbursed and the other 30 percent are a tax-deductible expense. The effective cost to the doctor of paying a good salary is miniscule. Also, if at any time any employed staff, from receptionists to nurses, are asked to take on added responsibilities, then some extra reward should also be forthcoming: a present if the extra responsibility is temporary, a payrise if it is permanent. This makes people realise that their efforts are appreciated and will encourage them to try even harder in the future.

TAKING ON NEW STAFF

Selection and employment of new staff is a hazardous undertaking, with many pitfalls for the unwary. Helpful guidelines can be obtained, by BMA members, from the BMA.

Drawing up a clear job description

A clear job description should be presented to every candidate for a post in the practice (see p. 202). This serves two purposes. First, the partners must sit down and look at the job and decide exactly what is needed. Unless employers have clear ideas about what they want their staff to do, the staff themselves are unlikely to be clear about what is expected of them. This does not engender a feeling of security.

Second, if the job description is well and thoroughly thought out, there can be no misunderstandings in the future about what the employee can reasonably be asked to do. Hopefully one should be able to avoid the kind of situation that forced a GP to write to the BMA asking for advice on how to deal with the receptionist who insisted that it was his job to make the morning coffee and not hers.

Though a job description is desirable, it is not a legal requirement. However, a contract of employment is. It should set out all the major particulars of employment, including the starting date, pay, hours, leave, sick pay, holidays, notice and grievance and disciplinary procedures. Employees are entitled to this information, and it is withheld at the employer's peril.

Selecting carefully

Before any interviews take place, there should be a consensus of opinion as to what qualities are being sought in the new member of staff. The views of those likely to be most affected should be given due weight. A 27-year-old secretary might well want to work with a colleague of around her own age or younger, and might feel threatened if an older, more powerful personality was going to be appointed. Some discussion before candidates are selected for interview helps to avoid this kind of problem.

One person — normally the practice manager or senior receptionist — should organise the mechanics of the proceedings, but the actual selection should be a joint effort. At least two or three people should be involved in the interviewing in order to minimise the possibilities of personality clashes. One of the interviewers should be someone who is going to work closely with the candidate.

TRAINING CONSCIENTIOUSLY

Every job needs some degree of skill and knowledge, and it is unfair for anybody to be expected to work without help or training. Before a new member of staff starts working, careful thought must be given to what is needed in the way of training and who the most appropriate people are to provide it.

Unless job training is planned in advance, the poor newcomer will have to learn on the job simply 'by watching Nellie'. The inevitable mistakes can be very demoralising and can retard progress. Structured training allows confidence to develop quickly — both in the worker who appreciates that the job is thought of highly enough to warrant the effort, and in the employer who can then be sure that the risk of unexpected disaster has been minimised.

PROVIDING ATTRACTIVE WORKING CONDITIONS

An employer's responsibilities do not end after selection and training. Staff welfare must be a priority, as happy and contented staff make for a happy and efficient practice.

Surgery accommodation should be warm, comfortable and well ventilated. A good rule of thumb would be to consider if you would be happy to work under the same conditions. If so, fine. If not, a few pounds spent on decorations or heating might make all the difference.

Volume of work must also be monitored to ensure that no-one is subjected to intolerable levels of stress. Managing a waiting room during surgery hours can be a hectic business and the doctor, insulated in the consulting room, may not be fully aware of what is going on. There should always be enough people for the job in hand and there should be time for relaxation and the all-important tea break.

Pay levels should be reviewed every year. It might be convenient to do this when the doctors get their own pay rises, and perhaps the staff deserve at least as much of a rise as their masters. For those loyal employees who stay with the practice for some time, there should be generous provision for holidays and sick pay. Full-timers, or even some of the part-timers, may deserve some pension provisions. This does not cost the doctor a lot, but is a valuable way of demonstrating appreciation for services rendered.

Adequate insurance cover should be secured, as an employer may be held responsible for accidents or injuries sustained at work.

Finally, the practice manager or one identified partner should be responsible for staff relationships, so that this person can be approached by anyone who feels troubled. Every employee will have moans and groans or new ideas about the job which need to be expressed. It helps knowing exactly whom to talk to when upset. Natural inhibitions about criticising the doctors have to be overcome and thoughts put into words. A recognised channel for complaint prevents any smouldering discontent and allows problems to be resolved more easily.

Making the most of receptionists

Practice receptionists must be one of the most unjustly maligned groups of people in society. Often described as dragons or battle-axes, they have acquired an image that is difficult to eradicate. Their predicament is mainly due to the fact that they are in the impossible position of having to satisfy the demands of the patients while at the same time having to comply with the instructions of their employers. Their freedom of action is often severely restricted by the time their doctors make available for consulting or the willingness of their doctors to do home visits.

When a patient is thwarted, it is usually regarded as the fault of the receptionist rather than the responsibility of the employer, the doctor. Patients therefore feel free to vent their anger and frustration on the receptionist, though they are usually very careful not to alienate the doctor. The same patient who has just finished being rude and aggressive in the waiting room is very likely to be all sweetness and light once in the consulting room.

It is the doctor's responsibility to employ staff of the right calibre and to give them adequate resources to do a good job.

LOOKING FOR DESIRABLE QUALITIES

A receptionist needs many qualities to be able to cope with the hurly-burly of a busy surgery. Primarily, she should be interested in and care for people. This is essential if she is to be able to listen to people patiently, to be tolerant of difficult behaviour and to understand inarticulate attempts at communication. This compassion needs to be married to maturity and sufficient inner steel to be able to be objective enough to withstand manipulative behaviour.

The ideal part-timer is therefore an intelligent woman who has had her family and has some experience of the problems of life. Having a mature appearance and being articulate helps patients to accept guidance and support. Most importantly, as she will have to work in a team, she will have to get on well with other people — particularly women.

Selection is therefore very important, and as many candidates as possible should be interviewed. There is an argument in favour of not having employees who are also patients. There are times when there may be a conflict of interests, and it may be fairer to the receptionist if she is not obliged to consult about a personal or embarrassing problem. Some patients may also be a bit worried if a local person they know has access to their medical records, though in rural areas it may be quite impossible to have an outsider, and the receptionists will have to be seen to be exceptionally discreet and reliable.

EDUCATING CONTINUOUSLY

In spite of the increasing complexities of reception work (see p. 193) there is very little in the way of formal training for the person who wants to make this a career. Some colleges of further education do run courses for medical secretaries, but these are heavily orientated towards secretarial and office skills. The newly recruited receptionist really has to be trained within the practice though, at present, for most this means they will receive very little other than on-the-job instruction. The GPs themselves generally actively avoid teaching, leaving this to the practice manager or to the other office staff.

As it is so unreasonable to expect anyone to perform well without training, every practice should make some effort to provide teaching for their receptionists. The new recruit will need basic instruction about the way in which the surgery is organised and quite a lot of new information about such things as certificates, appointments, taking calls and requests for repeat prescriptions.

Constructing a syllabus

A new member of staff may feel awkward about having to keep asking the others questions, particularly when they are busy. There is no guarantee that they will ask the right questions, get the right answers, or even that they will eventually gain all the information relevant to their job.

To make the initiation period less traumatic, and to ensure that every important topic is adequately covered, a simple syllabus should be constructed and one or two people delegated to be the 'official' teachers. Of course, all the nuts and bolts of reception work will have to be included, but by exercising a little imagination the scope of the enterprise can be fruitfully extended.

For example, there should be an opportunity to learn more about the care of patients and about how important the receptionist's role is in providing a friendly and effective service. Also some discussions should be aimed at improving verbal and interpersonal skills to enhance communications with patients, however difficult they are.

Arranging teaching sessions

After the receptionists have acquired the basic tools of the trade, occasional, but regular, teaching sessions should be arranged to allow them to satisfy their curiosity about such matters as the meaning and significance of presenting symptoms; how to assess the urgency of a case; how the commonly used drugs work and the conditions they are most likely to be used in; and how illness may affect the emotions and behaviour of patients.

These sessions should not be didactic talks but rather unstructured tutorials where interruptions and questions are actively encouraged. For most practices they will be purely internal affairs, but there is no reason why groups of practices could not arrange cooperative teaching of their receptionists in the local postgraduate centre. In Essex the local RCGP faculty has held a number of very popular receptionist study days.

Teaching the skills of answering the telephone and of handling patients is difficult and has to be carried out in as tactful a way as possible. The most practical method is to use role play in small groups. This can be done live or by using audio or video tapes of simulated patient problems. Another method is actually to tape or video the receptionists in action and then to let them listen to or watch the results. We have not yet used this latter method ourselves, but others have and their receptionists have not been too disconcerted. With either role play or video work, one of the priorities is to show how the wrong words or the wrong tone of voice can put down or antagonise patients, while openings which offer help and sympathy will deflect anger and gain maximum patient cooperation.

All this educative activity may seem to represent an impossible strain on the practice. In fact, we are only talking about an hour or two a month — at the most. Divided among partners this is negligible, especially when compared with the enormous dividends in goodwill and improved performance that will result.

CLARIFYING RESPONSIBILITIES

Because they deal directly with the public, receptionists often have to make quite responsible decisions. This is not easy, even for those with adequate training. For those without such training or with employers who have never clearly told them the limits of the responsibility they are allowed to exercise, the difficulties are compounded. Some receptionists, despite their worries about their ability to cope, come to the conclusion that their employers expect them to make quite sophisticated judgments. Others, more dangerously, come to overrate their own abilities and start to make judgments about strictly clinical matters.

Subjecting receptionists to feelings of insecurity over not knowing exactly what they can or cannot do is quite unfair. All receptionists should have the benefit of some sort of protocol which makes it very clear when they should hand over a particular problem to a doctor or practice manager. For instance, it might be reasonable for the practice to agree that receptionists should never be in the position of refusing a request for a visit or an urgent appointment.

Giving telephone advice is another responsible task undertaken by virtually all receptionists. Once again, there should be clear guidelines about what advice should or should not be given. This then has to be linked with teaching about the significance of symptoms and the pitfalls that lie in wait for the overconfident adviser. If receptionists are to be allowed to tell patients what to do for mild diarrhoea, then they have to make a competent attempt to ascertain the severity of the problem and the presence or absence of other significant symptoms.

Partners must agree among themselves, and then with the receptionists, clear guidelines about the nature of their work and just what responsibilities they are to undertake. Once agreed, these decisions should be written down and a copy should be immediately available in the office for staff to refer to.

To be realistic, one cannot write a tome of complicated rules to cover every eventuality, and the receptionists have to be allowed some freedom of action. In spite of this, some written instructions will help to prevent misunderstandings.

SUPPORTING PROPERLY

As receptionists are in such a vulnerable position, they need a lot of support. They must be certain of getting the backing of their doctors when things go wrong. This does not mean that they are immune from criticism if they behave inappropriately, but it does mean that they should get all the help they need when faced with situations they cannot handle by themselves.

Every practice has its tiny minority of patients who try to manipulate the receptionists or who are downright rude and aggressive. The doctor or, at the least, the practice manager should undertake the task of trying to re-educate these characters. If they are allowed to get away with bad behaviour on one or two occasions, they are likely to make it a habit. Receptionists should have no inhibitions about telling the doctor about any unsavoury incidents and leaving it up to him or her to tackle the patient.

It is too easy to hide away in the security of the consulting room and never be aware of the stresses to which receptionists can be subjected. It can be most helpful to take the time now and then to stand unobtrusively in the office and to listen to what is going on. Coupled with regular checks on the appointment books, this will give a good idea of what the pressure of work is likely to be. Do not hide behind the defensive wall of your consulting room door, get out there onto the ramparts.

Like the rest of us, receptionists need to be shown that their efforts are appreciated. Appropriate compliments cost little and can be supplemented now and then by more tangible evidence of esteem. This can take the form of bonuses or social events. A Christmas party or a practice dinner or other outing can do a lot to maintain morale and promote commitment to the work of the practice. For the money-conscious, such events are actually tax deductible.

Maintaining lines of communication

The very real danger that receptionists may feel isolated and unsupported can be minimised by making sure that the lines of communication between them and the doctors are always open. Information and ideas must flow in both directions. A stream of instructions, rather than a dialogue, will stifle enthusiasm.

There must be a mechanism by which they can freely express their own ideas and grievances and, when necessary, they should not be inhibited from telling the doctors where they are going wrong. We can make life difficult for them in so many ways — starting surgery late, forgetting to sign prescriptions, asking patients to ring up at the wrong time for results, or generally just by being grumpy or miserable. Someone should always be prepared to sit down and listen when pressures build up.

There should be regular, though not too frequent, meetings between the staff and the doctors. It is a good idea if just one partner attends, as otherwise the meeting is likely to be dominated by the doctors and there will not be a true interchange of feelings. Plenty of notice should be given, so that the receptionists can discuss their problems among themselves beforehand.

Free and uninhibited communication is the keystone to success. Do not be deluded into believing that lots of informal cheery chats really allow problems and feelings to be brought into the open. They are certainly valuable in their own right, but the receptionists are usually too protective towards and overawed by their doctors, and so need to pluck up a lot of courage to confront them with an unpleasant problem. Chance cannot be relied on for good communications; only hard work will produce the best results.

Creating a role for secretaries and practice managers

In a small practice the office staff have to be flexible and prepared to turn their hand to a variety of jobs. Nurse/receptionists, receptionist/secretaries, receptionist/practice managers and even more complex hybrid jobs have to be filled. With bigger practices more specialisation is possible, and a really large group may have a practice manager, two or three secretaries, a filing clerk and a switchboard operator or telephonist, as well as the usual complement of receptionists and practice nurses.

However big the practice and however specialised it might be possible to make the staff, it is very important to maintain flexibility to ensure that everyone can still cope with a wide variety of tasks. Apart from the obvious advantage of always having competent cover during holidays or illness, it makes everyone's job that much more challenging and interesting. A couple of hours on the switchboard can be a welcome break from the reception area, and the telephonist will also enjoy her break filing or keeping the age-sex register up to date. Job descriptions must encompass this versatility.

A JILL OF ALL TRADES

Though the role of the practice secretary will be dictated by the requirements of her particular practice, for most work is likely to be largely or wholly secretarial in nature. This does not lessen the importance of making the job as interesting and responsible as possible, and every secretary should be brought into regular contact with patients (ours help in reception from time to time and organise the antenatal clinic each week — including weighing patients, testing urines and filling in cooperation cards). A feeling of being involved in active patient care motivates the secretary to learn more about the job and to feel personally responsible for helping people (see p. 204).

From the business point of view, it almost goes without saying that the secretary should be competent in medical shorthand and typing and capable of carrying out administrative tasks delegated by the doctors. She should establish links with secretaries in hospitals, postgraduate centres, social services and all the other organisations which the practice has to deal with. This facilitates the making of appointments, the organisation of meetings, phoning for test results, and above all it makes it easier for her to wheedle out services for patients when these are needed.

In addition, she should accumulate practice-relevant information about the plethora of organisations that may, at some time or other, be of some service to the patient. Names and addresses of everything from abortion clinics to self-help groups should be readily to hand, so that the doctor can refer the patient to the secretary in order to establish the necessary contact.

Finally, she should be able to organise her employers. An efficiently kept appointments' diary is vital, particularly if some of the doctors are involved in medico-political or postgraduate activities. Such a diary can help to avoid those embarrassing mix-ups and double bookings that afflict us all from time to time.

A CUT ABOVE THE OTHERS

The idea for practice managers (see p. 205) grew out of the realisation that good practice organisation made many time-consuming demands on the administrative and business management skills of the partners. In some practices such skills were in short supply, while in others, though the skills were present, the inclination to spend the time exercising them was not.

Thus, often by default, senior receptionists took on many of these tasks, until the managerial role became too big for a part timer to handle and demanded a full-time manager. Nowadays the range of tasks undertaken by practice managers varies considerably from practice to practice and reflects the interests of the partners and the extent to which they wish to divest themselves of administrative tasks.

Utilising personnel management skills

In all but the smallest of practices there is a lot of hassle and work involved in the everyday business of paying staff salaries, deducting tax, arranging holidays and making up rotas. A manager can relieve the doctors of this considerable burden, and can also take on the tasks of maintaining staff morale and sorting out any interpersonal problems that may arise.

Personnel management skills are therefore an important quality to be looked for when selecting a practice manager. He or she has to be able to supervise other people's work and maintain a reasonable level of discipline in the office. This has to be achieved with subtlety, so that everybody remains friends and retains enthusiasm for the job. A well-managed office has a happy, bustling atmosphere about it, and this feeling will be reflected in the efficient yet kind way in which the staff deal with the public.

For these reasons it may be inadvisable for a practice wanting to appoint a manager to promote unthinkingly the most senior receptionist. Unless it is clear that the other staff will accept her as a leader, it may be wiser to advertise and bring in a new person.

Supervising a routine organisation

A natural corollary of the staff management role is supervision of all the routine systems operated by the staff. The appointment system is one facet of practice organisation that is likely to give rise to problems. The practice manager should be able to monitor the day-to-day operation of the system, watching both for discrepancies between demand and supply and for inappropriate responses to the patients. A manager should have the confidence to take the initiative to sort out these situations, though being able to confer with a designated partner makes the job easier and less stressful.

Though the appointment system may take up the most time, other systems involving age–sex and diagnostic registers, repeat prescribing, practice statistics, follow-ups or screening programmes should also be the business of the practice manager. His or her role should not be confined to supervision, but initiative and innovation should be encouraged as part of the job. Given the opportunity to see other practices or to attend a practice manager's course, ideas can be brought back to the practice and feasibility studies can be presented to the partners. Initiative should always be encouraged even if at first some of the ideas may not seem all that useful. A few failures are not necessarily a disaster and help temper enthusiasm with realism.

The same principles apply to the management of clinics and other special services. Immunisation, well baby, cervical smears and hypertension clinics and practice screening programmes all need active management and continual thought about how to maximise their efficiency.

Accounting and generally administering

One tedious but vital job that can be delegated is day-to-day book-keeping. Some practitioners prefer their staff not to have access to information about their personal incomes, and a lot will depend on how professional and reliable the manager is considered to be. However, if this job is not delegated, a partner or outside accountant will have to do it. At the least, the practice manager can control the petty cash and systems for monitoring payments for such items as insurance medicals or private patients.

A related accounting function is the maintenance of accurate returns to the FPC for patient registration and claims for item-of-service fees. To maximise income this has to be done efficiently and may involve the administrator in nagging the partners to fill in the appropriate forms.

Another administrative task which a manager will fulfil is that of maintaining the practice premises and compliance with insurance and health and safety at work regulations. It is comforting to know that, if a sink blocks up or the central heating breaks down, it is the administrator who will be phoning round the plumbers, not you.

Communicating upwards, downwards and sideways

An efficient practice manager will be in constant touch with all the other staff as well as with the partners. He or she is therefore the ideal person formally to look after the whole problem of intrapractice communication. In a big practice especially, it is very easy for one or two partners or receptionists to be told something and to assume that everyone else knows as well. The manager can make a point of telling everyone and can even send round a regular broadsheet.

Good communications need some organisation. Meetings have to be arranged or memos sent round. This process may include people and organisations outside the practice. Hospital administrators, social services department staff, local council staff and drug company representatives are just some examples of those with whom we have to exchange information or meet and with whom the practice manager can maintain regular contact.

Helping to teach others

Like everybody else in the practice who is in a position of any authority, the practice manager should be involved in the business of teaching. New receptionists and clerks need help and instruction, though those aspects of the job which the manager might find it difficult to teach personally should be delegated to the doctors, an example of delegation upwards rather than downwards. Trainees can be passed in the other direction.

Teaching should not just be a nominal part of the manager's job, as an interest in and an ability to teach enhances relationships and bolsters authority and leadership.

Getting the best out of nurses

Nurses may be involved in the delivery of primary medical care in many ways. As DHA employees they may undertake patient care in their own right, acting independently of any doctor, or be in the curious position of accepting work and medical direction from GPs while remaining ultimately under the control of their own administrative departments. As directly employed practice nurses, they undertake patient care on behalf of the partners, who have undiluted responsibility for their actions and whose Defence Union will legally cover them when they are working under the doctor's instructions.

WORKING WITH DISTRICT NURSES

District nurses are primarily concerned with the provision of nursing services for patients in their own homes. They can also carry out duties in the surgery, if requested by the GP and if allowed to by their administrators.

The majority of district nurses are attached to practices and should therefore be able to identify with and develop loyalties to the practice's patients and doctors. Unfortunately, after more than two decades of experimenting with attachments, the level of cooperation achieved is still not always good and now some DHAs are even setting the clock back by reallocating their district nurses' work on a geographical basis.

Lack of effective teamwork may simply be due to the personalities of both the district nurse and the doctors, though it may also be the result of poor practice organisation, which makes it impossible for the nurse to work in the surgery or to meet the partners on a regular basis. Even when cooperation at practice level is good, the development of new methods of working can be inhibited by the nurses' hierarchy, who may actively resist all change. Sometimes this may be a justifiable reaction to protect employees from mindless or inappropriate delegation, though at other times it stems far more from prejudice and a complete inability to grasp the possibilities for expanding the role and increasing the status of district nurses.

Getting the best out of the district nurse must involve the GP in some extra work. Maximising the possibilities for delegation is not the sole objective of the exercise, as all that this achieves is a reduction in the GP's workload and an increase in the nurse's. This is not an objective that will be seen as equally desirable by everybody. Work to be delegated should be work that can be carried out more appropriately or efficiently by the district nurse. This may be work that is normally done by the GP or it may be 'new' work, providing a better and expanded service to patients.

Knowing how far one can go

Just how much and what kind of work can be delegated to the district nurse depends very much both on the interests and attitudes of the nurse herself and of the nursing officer who administers the service. Being responsible to the health authority, the nurse may refuse, or be ordered not to accept, certain tasks. The amount of work that can be delegated will also depend on the staffing/workload ratios and, while in some areas the district nurse may be able to have a substantial commitment of work in the surgery, elsewhere this will be deemed impossible because the nurses appear to be fully occupied looking after patients in their own homes.

Local attitudes, staffing levels and interpersonal relationships are therefore the factors which will determine just how well GPs and nurses will integrate their work. It is important to have a realistic assessment of just what is or is not possible and then to establish the best working relationship on that basis. This can best be achieved by making sure that both parties meet from time to time, other than fortuitously at a patient's bedside. Such meetings do not have to be formalised. If coffee, biscuits and a welcome are available at the practice at a regular time, contacts will become more frequent. Once a friendly relationship is established, discussions will reveal exactly what each party expects of the other and so make misunderstandings less likely.

Ask, don't order

Conflict may arise if the GP does not appreciate that the modern nurse sees herself as an independent professional. Thus one does not order a nurse to do something, but sends or refers a patient to a nurse for a particular purpose. If a practice wants a nurse to do jobs like taking blood samples or syringing ears, then this has to be negotiated and agreed before any referring takes place. Some district nurses are quite willing to take on new and interesting roles, but others shy away from taking any extra responsibility, especially if this involves any kind of clinical judgment. Whatever their views, and no matter how illogical they may seem, only their own nursing hierarchy has the authority to direct their labour.

Reasonable requests are most likely to be successful where the nurse concerned feels friendly towards and respected by the practice and where she knows that she will never be left without effective support or out of her depth.

DIRECTLY EMPLOYING PRACTICE NURSES

To escape from the limitations imposed by the present role of the district nurses and their employment by health authorities, GPs have begun to employ their own practice nurses in ever-increasing numbers. This allows greater flexibility, more control over practice-relevant activities and an increased level of delegation.

By directly employing nurses, the partners can choose people of more than adequate calibre and compatible personality. To achieve the best results they then have to be treated as fellow professionals and well paid at a rate commensurate with their responsibilities. Once the relationship is right, then can follow the training necessary to equip them fully for their mutually agreed role (see p. 197).

Delegating fairly

We have discussed the arguments for delegation earlier (see p. 123). Here we would just like to say that employment of a nurse does not carry with it an automatic right to delegate any kind of work to her. Equally for safety and for fairness, both parties have to agree that the nurse is fully competent to carry out the delegated task. From the doctor's viewpoint this means accepting the responsibility for training, teaching and supervising the nurse's work until, and after, a satisfactory level of competence is achieved. From the nurse's viewpoint it means not accepting tasks unless happy to do so and then only after enough training has taken place to give justifiable confidence in her own ability to cope unaided.

We are convinced that practice-employed nurses can play an increasingly responsible role in the delivery of primary care. With people of high calibre, maturity and experience, the possibilities are tremendous. The term Nurse Practitioner may be appropriate for this new breed of practice nurses. In our experience patients accept them readily — perhaps a little too readily for the the health of our egos!

LABOURING WITH THE COMMUNITY MIDWIVES

In many districts in recent years, community midwives have suffered major changes in their role and status. A generation ago, when domiciliary obstetrics was still normal practice in most areas, they were independent practitioners who took personal responsibility for the obstetric care of their patients. The move towards hospital obstetrics has meant that in many cases district midwives, like GPs, have been reduced to providing antenatal and postnatal care only.

GP obstetric units have allowed the retention of some intrapartum care, but strict selection criteria have considerably reduced the numbers for delivery. Even where there is a GP unit, large duty rotas mean that a patient is very unlikely to be actually delivered by the midwife she has seen antenatally.

Where a GP does undertake intrapartum care, the quality of the service very much depends on the quality and attitudes of the community midwives. As with district nurses, it is important to be realistic about what the local arrangements have to offer. If it is impossible to secure a reliable, personal and technically efficient service for practice patients from the midwives, then the practice ought to consider relinquishing the intrapartum care of their patients.

A midwife with energy and flexible attitudes is a tremendous asset to any practice. She should be persuaded to attend the practice antenatal clinics and, if a room is available, she could interview and advise patients at other times as well. Like the health visitors, midwives are always giving advice to patients, and it is therefore imperative that there is some agreement about how the patients are going to be managed during their pregnancies. When deliveries are being undertaken in a GP unit, there must be a clear understanding about what is regarded as normal progress during labour and when the GP is to be called. With efficient teamwork, this is a very satisfying aspect of practice, but when doctors and midwives cannot rely on each other, it can be a nightmare.

APPRECIATING OTHER SPECIAL ROLES

Clinic nurses

Clinic nurses are DHA employees who on the whole have little contact with GPs, as they are mainly concerned with the running of child surveillance clinics. The amount of further education needed to do this job is not great, so they are fairly low down the career structure and are paid at staff nurse rates.

Unfortunately, nurses employed in health centres by the DHA are, for historical reasons, also classified as clinic nurses. Though they often function as practice nurses and may take on quite a lot of responsible work, it may be very difficult to increase their salary to a level appropriate to their responsibilities.

Hospital-based community nurses

Specialised nurses such as community psychiatric nurses, community diabetic nurses and even community neurological nurses are comparative newcomers to the community scene. Though they operate in the community, they are based in specialised hospital departments and are charged with the follow-up of patients who have already been treated in the hospital. If communications with the GP are good, then the patient will benefit from the extra time and skills that are available. Where contact is minimal, there is a very real danger that the patient may suffer from conflicting and disorganised advice.

The practice can make best use of these nurses by ensuring that information about new events or changes in treatment is passed on to them. Communication in one direction should stimulate a flow in the reverse direction, and a useful dialogue should be established.

Where possible, it is worth attracting the nurses into the surgery by encouraging them to see mutual patients on the premises. Once a *de facto* attachment has been achieved, it is possible to involve them in the care of patients who have never been to the hospital. Diabetic nurses are usually quite happy to do blood sugar profiles on new diabetics who do not need referral; psychiatric nurses are often quite keen to start psychotherapy groups or to undertake behavioural desensitisation programmes for phobic patients. These activities enhance the professional identities of the nurses concerned, as well as giving practice patients a better service.

Cooperating with health visitors

Health visitors have to undertake quite a lot of training after they qualify as nurses, and consequently have an even more highly developed sense of professional identity than district nurses. Also, health visitor courses include a lot of sociology which leads them to take a generally jaundiced view of the traditionally dominant role of the doctor.

The same political forces that led to the attachment of nurses led to the widespread assignment of health visitors to individual practices. Attachment was not always welcomed unreservedly by either doctors or health visitors and, once again, success was determined very much by local attitudes and interpersonal relationships. Where there was mutual respect and liking, good working partnerships developed.

PARTNERSHIP RULES

Partnership is in fact a good word to describe the way GPs and health visitors should work together. Health visitors have both the skills and the time to provide an advisory and supervisory service to mothers with young children. This service should complement rather than supplant those provided by the GP.

Ideally, the health visitor should do most of her work in and from the practice premises. This will be automatically considered in the case of health centres, but other practices may well have to negotiate or even resort to low cunning to lure a health visitor into the surgery. If a health visitor is doing well-baby sessions from a nearby clinic, then the way to entice her into the surgery is by running a practice clinic which attracts so many patients that the DHA clinic becomes starved of custom. The health visitor will go where the patients are and will help the practice to provide an even better standard of care.

If a desirable health visitor is attracted, then the practice must ensure that she has the room and the facilities to do the job properly. This may cost some money, but the extra help will make it money well spent.

The exact role of the health visitor varies from area to area and from person to person. Some regard geriatric surveillance as part of their job, while others confine themselves very much to looking after children. There must be agreement about how they are going to coordinate their efforts with those of the practice. Discussions are essential to plan an effective service, e.g. one common interest is in maximising immunisation rates, and an agreed system for patient education and the chasing up of defaulters, together with access to practice records, will increase the chances of success.

SPEAKING WITH ONE VOICE

The health visitor has constant contact with patients and spends a lot of time giving them advice. It is therefore vital that doctors and health visitors are saying the same things in the same way. Conflicting advice or advice that can be interpreted in different ways can be very disruptive and may lead to ill-feeling. Patients may be confused or irritated, or they may make use of mismatched information in a manipulative way. Partners and health visitors must take the time and the trouble to agree common policies for simple everyday problems. This may sound an easy thing to do, but it is surprising how often ill-feeling about differing approaches exists while no-one has taken any initiative to start discussions to evolve common policy. Talking regularly should be part of any working relationship and, once instituted, will quickly resolve existing differences.

A mature and capable health visitor can be a tremendous asset in any practice. Apart from the routine services she provides, she may also be well placed to counsel women patients with emotional or marital problems. She should know a lot about, and be skilled in, mobilising other services which may be of use to patients, e.g. Gingerbread groups, mother and baby clubs and the Marie Curie fund.

By talking to your health visitors and treating them with respect, you can make sure that your patients will benefit from their expertise.

All aboard the 'S.S. Caritas'

A prime practice function is to direct patients appropriately to other professionals or agencies who can provide useful services, which otherwise might not be available. When lack of skill, time or inclination conspire to leave a gap in the practice's service, then there is a clear duty to try and fill the gap by utilising someone else's talents.

There may also be, in certain circumstances, an equally clear duty to protect patients from the inappropriate or harmful attentions of confidence tricksters — medical and lay — who seek to take advantage of ignorance and gullibility.

APPRECIATING SOCIAL WORKERS

Social workers, the profession that was created almost overnight by Seebohm, are a neglected and much-maligned group. This is unfortunate, as a good working relationship with the local social services department can pay handsome dividends. Once again, actually talking to someone increases the chances of understanding and cooperation developing. A meeting or two, perhaps over lunch, with the local director of social services or the area team leader can often be the start of a fruitful relationship.

A frequent cause of resentment among social workers is the difficulty they have in getting to talk to GPs about mutual clients. The combination of defensive receptionists and unenthusiastic doctors often defeats attempts at communication and produces a feeling of rejection. Courtesy and a demonstrable willingness to talk should improve relationships and help to get a better service for the practice's patients.

Whenever possible, invite the local social worker round to the surgery. Once the habit of dropping in has been developed, it may become regularised by custom and develop into an 'unofficial' attachment. This approach can work in a practice where official requests for attachments have been turned down for economic or political reasons. The social worker's role in the practice can be more firmly established if he or she is allowed to use one of the consulting rooms to interview mutual clients.

This 'softlee, softlee, catchee monkee' approach can also be used to draw other people with useful talents into the web of primary care. Marriage guidance counsellors are a good example.

BEING PRAGMATIC ABOUT FRINGE PRACTITIONERS

Whether their doctors like it or not, many patients go to see fringe practitioners. This can be somewhat ego-denting, and traditionally we do not sully our virginal professional status by consorting with such outsiders. However, instead of maintaining a sterile air of disdain, it might be better to take the trouble to find out just what they have to offer. By keeping eyes and ears open it is relatively easy to discover which osteopaths, hypnotists and what have you practise in a responsible fashion and when exactly their services are likely to be of value.

Patients often refer themselves, without risking asking their doctor's opinion. Some, however, want to know if a particular treatment will be likely to help them and deserve a fairly open-minded reply. Their enquiries are usually only made when conventional therapy has failed and, provided there are no grounds for believing that alternative medicine will cause them any harm, it is not unreasonable to point them in the direction of someone known to be above-board. This is better than allowing them to forage for themselves and risk falling into some chareatan's clutches.

Of course, further enquiries into fringe disciplines might lead to attendance at lectures, demonstrations or courses, and hypnosis, acupuncture and manipulation might well become additional strings to the practice's bow. Useful additional services might then be provided to practice or private patients or, at the least, far more appropriate selection of patients for referral will be achieved.

BEING EQUALLY PRAGMATIC ABOUT PRIVATE PRACTITIONERS

When patients make a reasonable request to be referred to another practitioner privately for a second opinion then, however annoying this may sometimes be, their wishes should be explored and met. The doctor's political or moral beliefs should not be imposed on the patients and, as a trusted adviser, the GP should give objective advice and acquiesce to reasonable requests.

When patients go directly to another doctor privately then, in theory, that doctor should ask the GP's permission before the consultation takes place. In very few cases nowadays is this ethical courtesy actually adhered to, and the best the GP is likely to get is a letter beginning 'Your patient attended me today, but unfortunately forgot to bring your letter' or 'Thank you for referring this patient, whom I saw without benefit of your letter of introduction'. In this kind of situation the GP has every right to take the patient and the doctor — especially the doctor — to task.

Unfortunately, prostituting one's normal behaviour and standards for money is an undesirable trait which some doctors possess in a highly developed form. While care must be taken about ever criticising another doctor's actions, there is a moral imperative to protect patients from the minority of private practitioners, consultants or fellow GPs, who are trying to exploit them. One good example is the 'Slimmers' Clinic' which dispenses appetite suppressants and diuretics to patients at exorbitant prices. Such patients should be told in no uncertain terms that they are being conned.

On the other hand, some private practitioners may be able to offer a useful service to patients, having time and skills that perhaps you do not possess. Fellow GPs may, for instance, do vasectomies or be particularly good at hypnosis or psychotherapy, and it may be more convenient for a patient to see them rather than go through a NHS referral process.

DON'T FORGET YOUR LOCAL PARAMEDICAL BUSINESS-PEOPLE

Friendly relations with the local chemists cost nothing and may well pay dividends in the form of unsolicited oral testimonials. They may also help to avoid potential prescribing disasters when illegible or inaccurate scripts are presented. The least courtesy which should be extended to all chemists is immediate telephone access to the doctor. Any script query should be dealt with straight away to lessen the risk of a wrong formulation being impatiently dispensed or a patient leaving before the script is actually made up.

Good relations with the local opticians and undertakers are also worth maintaining. In the optician's case, easy access of practice patients to a tonometer is one valuable benefit.

Section 5
Nuts and Bolts

Introduction

This section is intended to provide a framework round which ideas for running a practice may be arranged. The style is not intended to be discursive and in parts may seem to be just a succession as headlines. A good newspaper editor will say, however, that the reader should be able to get the gist of any articles solely by reading the headlines, though hopefully he or she will then be seduced into reading on.

Practice premises

A good practice needs premises that are large enough for comfort, are efficient in use and are pleasant to work in. The cost-rent scheme and rent and rate rebates have brought adequate premises within the financial reach of every practice. If you are thinking of building new premises or upgrading old ones:

1. Visit practices that have recently gone through the same experience.
2. Invest time and effort on research and design.
3. Use an architect who has experience of planning premises for GPs.
4. Consider asking the advice of the Medical Architecture and Research Unit, Holloway, London N7 8DB.

When you are drawing up specifications or looking at plans, ask yourself about:

Accessibility Is there adequate car parking for patients, including the disabled, and the practice team?

Disabled people Has provision been made for ramps, lifts and other aids?

Toilets Are there adequate toilet facilities?

Corridors Is there room for prams and wheelchairs to get about? Do you want prams in the corridors — if not, is there a secure and covered pram park?

Comfort Is the building well lit and easy to maintain? Is the atmosphere relaxing and welcoming?

Confidentiality Can patients talk to receptionists without being overheard? Are the consulting rooms soundproof? NB: No communicating door is soundproof.

Office There must be planty of room for filing, staff and future expansion. Are there separate rooms for the secretary and practice manager?

Workspace Is there room for all the present and possible future members of the team? If there is space for their nurses, social workers, psychologists and so on may all want to work with you.

Is there somewhere for doctors and staff to sit, talk and drink coffee away from the public gaze? Can staff enter and leave the premises without going through the waiting room?

Layout Do patients have easy access to the consulting room from the waiting room? Can the receptionists keep an eye on the waiting room? Is the patient call system efficient?

Are the premises expandable and adaptable for future needs?

CONSULTING ROOM LAYOUT

The way a surgery is laid out can have a substantial effect on the dynamics of the consultation. It can also tell you a lot about the personality and consulting style of the doctor.

The desk

This is the largest and most important item of office furniture, and its position in relation to the doctor and the patient is central in determining whether the consultation will be doctor or patient-orientated.

Traditional The doctor faces the patient across the desk (Fig. 5.1).
1. Preserves the authority of the doctor and enhances his or her control of the consultation.
2. Does not allow mobility.
3. Discourages touching.
4. The doctor can isolate the patient further by cluttering the space on the desk between them with equipment, papers etc.

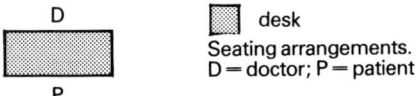

Seating arrangements.
D = doctor; P = patient

Fig. 5.1

Open Doctor and patient sit side by side near a desk or do away with the desk altogether (Fig. 5.2).
1. Decreases the doctor's authority.
2. Reduces barriers and encourages mobility and touching.
3. Enforced intimacy may actually reduce the level of verbal communication.

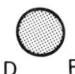

Fig. 5.2 Seating arrangements; D = doctor; P = patient

Accessible Doctor and patient sit near each other across the corner of the desk (Fig. 5.3).
1. Patient easily accessible.
2. Reduces barriers and encourages mobility and touching.
3. Patient not forced into intimacy — privacy is respected.
4. Verbal interaction is maximal in this position.

For further information read the chapter by Patrick Pietroni 'Nonverbal Communication in the general practice surgery' in Bernice Taumer (ed) 'Language and Communication in General Practice'

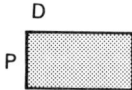

Fig. 5.3

The appointment system

This section is intended to provide a framework round which ideas for running an appointment system may be arranged. The appointment system should spread the workload evenly through the week, reduce the waiting time for patients, avoid overcrowding in the waiting room, and give the doctor the ability to plan the week's work. It should not make it more difficult for patients to see their doctor, or prevent people who genuinely feel that their problem is urgent from being seen the same day. Routine or non-urgent appointments should be available with the doctor of choice within 24–72 hours, though not necessarily at the exact time of the patient's choosing.

The sick appointments system is one where demand consistently outstrips supply, so that patients are forced to wait for excessive periods before being seen. Disillusionment and agression may build up in the practice, with receptionists being put under unecessary stress and the doctors seeing themselves as being overworked.

The treatment must be to increase the number of appointments available while long-term plans to modify demand or delegate work are put into effect.

PLANNING A SYSTEM

The number of consultations per patient per year varies from 1.6 to 6 and averages out at about 3.5. For a practice where each doctor looks after 2250 patients, each doctor will need to provide 8375 appointments annually. Allowing for holidays, this means 182 apointments weekly. Assuming nine sessions per week, this means 20 appointments per surgery.

A doctor who is away for an extra half day a week for leisure or other work will lose 920 appointments a year. The number seen per session multiplied by the number of sessions must equal the need! Where a system is overloaded, try adding three or four appointments to each and every surgery. This may make all the difference.

Flexibility is necessary, as demand does fluctuate. However, patients who need to be seen have to be seen sooner or later and postponing the event does nothing to lessen the load.

The availability of appointments should be monitored each day, either by a partner or the practice manager or senior receptionist. If demand is beginning to outstrip the supply, then he or she should have the power to increase each surgery by 15–30 minutes. If this is still not enough to maintain the service, then all partners should be 'requested' to fit in an extra surgery at some convenient time during the week. This situation should only really arise if a partner is suddenly withdrawn from service by illness or some other unforeseen crisis.

A further buffer can be provided by having a duty doctor who does a surgery which is not booked until that day. This will only work in a group practice where lists are allowed to mix. Where lists are adhered to, the same effect can be achieved by always keeping a few appointments unbooked in each surgery until the day.

Continuity of service can be maintained by staggering consulting hours throughout the day. Keeping the surgery open most of the time also evens out the workload and gives patients better access. Having a duty doctor for the day who is readily available allows the partners to get on with their routine work, provides a more rapid response to emergencies and gives moral support to the receptionists.

Safeguards should be built into the system, and receptionists should never be allowed to refuse an appointment or even actively to dissuade the patient from coming. Prescriptions should not be offered as an alternative, and a close eye should be kept on what is going on in the reception area.

Receptionist training

Patients' opinions about the practice are considerably influenced by the way they have been managed by the receptionists. They have an important and difficult job, and deserve all the help they can get to improve their performance.

BENEFITS OF TRAINING

1. Improves knowledge and skills. Increased efficiency helps patients and the practice.
2. Improves attitudes. Helps receptionists to understand patients' problems, making them kinder and more able to withstand difficult behaviour.
3. Gives professional pride and confidence.
4. Engenders feeling of being an important part of the team.
5. Improves the status of receptionists, hopefully leading to better pay and conditions.

METHODS OF TRAINING

1. *'Sitting with Nellie'':* learning by observation and example. Essential — but slow. Does not do much to help understanding.
2. *One-to-one teaching:* by senior receptionist, practice manager or the GP. Useful for rapid factual input and for discussions about problem-solving.
3. *Reading:* Pulse Blue Book and the DHSS Receptionist's Handbook are essential. Many of the articles in the weekly journals such as Pulse and GP are useful. Cut them out and file in the

office for reference.
4. *Group discussions:* Group teaching sessions. These can be organised on an intrapractice basis or can be run on a cooperative basis for neighbouring practices. Helpful to be able to meet and exchange ideas with other practices.
5. *Video or tape recording:* a bit threatening, but very useful for changing behaviour.
6. *Role playing:* a good way to practise telephone answering techniques or the responses to patients at reception.
7. *Using a special Modified Essay Question:* this can be given to individuals or more usefully discussed in a group.
8. *Extended courses:* run by polytechnics or similar institutions. Not many available. Sometimes difficult for part-timers to attend. Very useful for those taking on the role of practice manager.
9. *Exchange visits* to other practices. Informative and very popular with receptionists.

Sample patient management questionaire

Each episode is printed on a successive sheet of paper so that the answers to one episode are not affected by knowledge about what happens next.

Question 1 At 11.00 a.m., just as your surgery is finishing, a tired-looking woman (Mrs Young) with three small children comes to the reception desk and asks if she can sign on with the doctor. Your doctor's list is not full and he is accepting new patients. Mrs Young says that she has moved house recently. How do you deal with her?

Question 2 Mrs Young offers you three rather tatty medical cards which belong to herself and two of the children. You also notice that the doctor's name on the cards is that of a GP who works close by. What do you do?

Question 3 When you finish telling her about signing on, she asks if she can see the doctor now, as one of the children is not very well. How do you handle this?

Question 4 Some weeks later at the end of evening surgery, Mrs Young rings up and asks for a visit for her youngest child, who is about one year old and has had diarrhoea and vomiting for two days. What do you ask her and what do you do?

Question 5 You do not hear from the family again until one morning when Mr Young turns up in the surgery at 10.30 a.m. and says that he wants to see the doctor. You have an appointment system and there are no appointments left for that morning (the surgery ends at 10.45). What do you say to him?

Question 6 Mr Young appears to have only a mild cold and looks quite well. He insists that he needs a certificate today, and if the doctor will not see him now he will call him out. What is your next move?

Question 7 Your doctor is rather annoyed by Mr Young's attitude and declines to see him immediately, but he is offered an appointment for the evening surgery. Mr Young is not at all pleased. He tells the waiting room at large that this is a bloody useless surgery and you need to be dying before the doctor will see you. He then crashes out of the surgery. Do you do anything?

Question 8 Six months later, Mrs Young rings us just as your doctor is starting the evening surgery and says that her youngest child is having a fit. What do you do?

Question 9 Mr Young comes one evening for the medical for an HGV licence. He is 15 minutes early. The doctor, on the other hand, is half an hour behind with his appointments (not an unusual occurrence with this particular doctor). Do you do anything about this? There are still five other patients waiting to see him, besides Mr Young.

Question 10 A month later Mrs Young comes in for an appointment. She looks very run-down. When she comes out of the surgery she is in tears and tells you that Dr Jones has been very sharp with her and asks if she could please see another doctor in future. Dr Jones appears to have been in a bad temper all morning! How do you help Mrs Young?

Question 11 Dr Jones goes on being bad-tempered with staff and patients during the next few weeks. If there anything you can do?

Question 12 At Christmas Mrs Young comes in with a big box of chocolates for the staff. Why do you think she did this? Do you feel guilty?

Study days for receptionists

These sample programmes have all been used at several postgraduate centres and have all been very well received. The same subjects can be used on an intrapractice basis if the programme is broken down into smaller units.

Study day 1

10.00 a.m.	Films on practice management (Parke-Davis).
10.30 a.m.	*Coffee*
11.00 a.m.	Forms. The general practice. Organisation. Correct use.
12.00	Appointments systems. Reasons for such. Flexibility. Efficient organisation.
1.00 p.m.	*Lunch*
2.00 p.m.	Group work using patient management questionaire.
3.00 p.m.	Plenary session.
4.00 p.m.	*Tea*

Study day 2

10.15 a.m.	*Coffee*
10.30 a.m.	Symptoms. Important symptoms and their significance.
11.30 p.m.	Basic first aid.
12.30 p.m.	Practice mouth-to-mouth resuscitation with doll.
1.00 p.m.	*Lunch*
2.00 p.m.	Group work with patient management questionaire.
3.30 p.m.	Plenary session.
4.00 p.m.	*Tea*

Study day 3

10.15 a.m.	*Coffee*
10.30 a.m.	Common drugs used in general practice. Uses and dangers.
11.30 a.m.	How illness affects a patient. Social and emotional effects. Understanding behaviour.
12.30 p.m.	The rules of prescribing. Pharmacist.
1.00 p.m.	*Lunch*
2.00 p.m.	Group work with patient management questionaire.
3.30 p.m.	Plenary session.
4.00 p.m.	*Tea*

The content of these sessions should not be limited to the basic information that is necessary for the job. Most receptionists are very keen to learn more about patients and their problems. This makes the job more interesting and increases their understanding of how patients are affected by illness.

Practice nurses

One of the biggest changes in practice in the last decade or so has been the increasing number of nurses employed.

The advantages of employing practice nurses are:

* A better service can be provided for the patients, as nursing procedures, e.g. injections, dressings, are done on the premises.
* The doctor can delegate work — the time saved can be used for other purposes.
* As 70 per cent of salaries are reimbursed, the extra help in the practice costs very little.
* A nurse directly employed by the doctor has the work of the practice, particularly that in the surgery, as her first priority.
* Better preventative medicine can boost practice income by increasing item-of-service payments. The practice can then become both more cost-effective and medically efficient.
* Patients will occasionally air a problem which they perceive as too trivial to 'worry' a doctor with, but which does have clinical significance.
* Patients can see the nurse without an appointment.

THE WORK OF A PRACTICE NURSE

This can be divided into two main categories:

1. Nursing duties — work that is traditionally done by a nurse and for which more training will not be required.
2. Paramedical or medical work — duties which are less likely to be regarded as normal for a nurse and for which special training is needed. Some of this work is traditionally regarded as being that of a doctor.

1. Nursing duties

* General supervision of medical stores, drugs and instruments. Stock control, ordering. Sterilising.
* Routine dressings, injections, ear syringing.
* Simple advice to patients — in person or on the telephone about minor ailments or trauma.
* Taking of pathology specimens, including bloods

2. Paramedical or medical work

* Immunisation.
* Diagnostic procedures — ECGs, allergy testing, blood sugars Hbs, ESRs, uring tests, peak flow.
* Screening procedures, BP, cervical smears, breast examinations.
* Family planning — advice, cap fittings, routine checks for pill and coils.
* Diets — advice for obesity, diabetics, etc.
* Follow-up of chronics — patients stablished, i.e. hypertension, cardiac failure, disabled. At home or in the surgery.
* Follow-up of acute cases. Patients seen by doctor — single follow-up to check progress.
* Primary contact with patients. Consultations for minor ailments, rashes, sore throats, etc. — at home or in the surgery.

ADMINISTRATION

* Nurse must be given adequate room and facilities.
* Salary — should be generous, at least that of a ward sister of similar experience. Seventy per cent reimbursed by FPC but level of salary must be negotiated with them before employment, not after.
* Pension — consider providing a pension.
* Contract — a contract must be given. This should specify salary scales, pension arrangements, sick leave, study leave and notice to be given. The nature of the duties and training should be specified.
* Coordination — the district nurse must be kept informed about the nature of the practice nurses' duties. Work can overlap and friction must be avoided if at all possible. Try to arrange regular meetings of all nursing staff.

* RCN — the practice should pay for RCN membership, as this is the nurses' representative professional body.
* Arrangements for transport costs — use of a car for visits.

NURSE TRAINING

* No work should be delegated unless the nurse has been adequately trained. The nurse and the doctor must agree that the training has been adequate. The nurse must agree that the work being delegated is appropriate.
* Training for a specific function — must include theoretical and practical work before the nurse can be asked to function by herself. This programme must be formalised and there should be strict practice policies about what should be delegated. When these functions are identified, appropriate training must be organised.

At all times the nurse should feel free to ask for advice, a revisit or reassessment from the doctor without any hindrance or hint of annoyance from the doctor.

If she is at all worried, this must not be looked on as failure or incompetence.

CRITERIA FOR SELECTION OF A NURSE TO CARRY OUT PARAMEDICAL FUNCTIONS

Few nurses, by training or inclination, are suited to this job.

Qualifications

1. Mature persons with older family.
2. Used to responsibility, i.e. ex-theatre sister or casualty sister.
3. Heaps of common sense, plus a sense of adventure.
4. Enthusiasm for the job.

SAMPLE TRAINING PACKAGES BY GPs FOR SPECIFIC FUNCTIONS

Measles

A nurse should not be asked to do a primary or a follow-up visit for measles until:

* She has been given theoretical instruction about the pathology, clinical features and natural history of the common infective illnesses. Differential diagnosis and possible complications must be discussed.
* Specific features which the nurse should look for must be identified.
* She has the practical skills to examine the ears, throat and chest.
* There are clear guidelines for referral to the doctor laid down.
* She has been taken to see cases of measles by the doctor — for practical instruction.
* She feels confident to manage by herself.

Hypertension

A hypertensive should not be handed over for follow-up unless:

* There has been adequate theoretical instruction about the nature, natural history and treatment of hypertension.
* The nurse has clear cut instructions about what parameters have to be noted — e.g. BP, pulse, breathing, peripheral circulation and Us and Es, ECG where appropriate.
* The nurse knows what symptoms to enquire about, e.g. breathlessness, pains in the chest.
* A clear-cut protocol for follow-up is established, e.g. patient seen three times a year by the nurse and once a year by the doctor.
* There is a clear protocol for reference back to the doctor, e.g. rise in BP, new symptoms.

TRAINING BY OTHER AGENCIES

Nurses can be trained for specific functions by a variety of other people — this has to be negotiated by the GP.

* Diets — the area dietician.
* ECG — hospital electrocardiographer.
* Family planning — regional health authorities organise programmes for family planning nurses, which are very good value.
* Allergy testing — training will be done by representatives of companies wanting to sell desensitising vaccine, e.g. Bencard, Dome.

CONTINUING EDUCATION

Regular programmes of seminars for all nursing staff are essential. This maintains standards and morale and allows the exchange of views and information. In a big practice these may be entirely informal affairs. Smaller practices could arrange meeting on a cooperative basis.

LEGAL PROBLEMS

Many general practitioners are worried about the legal difficulties inherent in delegation of work.

1. For purely nursing duties — cover is provided by RCN membership.
2. For other delegated work — we have taken advice from the MDU and the principles are:
   a. Training must be adequate and preferably documented.
   b. Agreement has to be reached between doctor and nurse that the delegation is appropriate.

Under these conditions, the doctor is responsible and the consequences of the nurse's actions are covered by the doctor's MDU membership.

COMMUNICATIONS

* Good communications are essential.
* Nurses — attached or directly employed should have regular meetings with the doctors to discuss policy and for training.
* The nurses must feel that they have *free* access to the doctor for advice and that they can at *any* time refer patients back. This is absolutely essential and they must never feel inhibited about it.
* District nurses and practice nurses should liaise regularly to avoid misunderstandings and any demarcation problems, though if the district nurses are hostile and do not wish to be involved with the practice activities, then services should continue to evolve with the hope that they might 'come round' later.

Preparing a job description

When employing staff, it is essential to offer them an accurate job description. Although that may be a time-consuming exercise, it has the added benefit of identifying the exact nature of the job in the doctor's mind — a useful bonus when considering what exactly a new receptionist is being employed for.

A pragmatic solution is to write down the following list of headings on the left-hand side of the page and fill in the answers accordingly.

FOR A CLERICAL ASSISTANT

TITLE OF POST	Full-time clerical assistant.
RESPONSIBLE TO	Health centre administrator.
REPORTS TO	The administrator.
CONDITIONS OF SERVICE	Whitley Council for the Health Services (Great Britain) Clerical and Administrative Staff.
PLACE OF WORK	The health centre.
HOURS OF DUTY	37 hours per week — Monday to Friday.
GRADE	Scale II.
SCOPE OF WORK	To act as clerk/receptionist in the office. Duties will include typing, clerical, reception, filing, switchboard, etc., day-to-day work being allocated by the Administrator.
DUTIES Typing	* Assist medical secretaries as required.

	* Non-confidential work for the administrator.
	* New cards for persons registering.
	* Prepare and distribute weekly bulletin.
Stationery	* Maintain and order stocks, furnish offices, and stock cupboards. Check incoming supplies.
Relief	* Provide regular relief as arranged; assist in treatment room clerical work, cover staff shortages.
Assist	* Telephone operator with clerical duties.
Post	* Prepare and dispatch daily — complete record card.
Lunches	* Seminars, GP's meetings; order, arrange and prepare as necessary.
Ambulances	* Book by letter or telephone — deal with enquiries.
Follow-up book	* Check and send for patients regularly.
Filing	Maintain administrators' files.
OTHER WORK	* To be undertaken for other people or department only with the approval of the administrator.
	* May be modified after discussion with post-holder.
	* Any other task that may be found appropriate.
TRAINING	Will be given as necessary.

Before finally hiring someone, take up references and take advice whether the post is exempt from the provisions of the Rehabilitation of Offenders Act. This is particularly relevant where someone working in the NHS has access to confidential records, money or drugs.

FOR A RECEPTIONIST

The exact nature of a receptionist's job will vary from practice to practice, depending on local conditions and the organisational whims of the GPs. In a small practice the receptionist may well have to take on the roles of a secretary or a practice manager, while in the larger establishment the jobs are more likely to be specialised.

Whatever the nature of the practice, it is important that the receptionists have a clear and agreed idea of what the job entails. Staff have a right to a job description, so every practice should sit down and write out one that suits their particular circumstances. This exercise clarifies ideas and helps to prevent misunderstandings.

A sample description of the duties might be:

* Receptionists will receive instructions from and be responsible to the practice manager.
* Open and prepare the promises for work in the morning. Lock up and secure the premises at night.
* Prepare and tidy consulting rooms, including stocking up with stationery.
* Receive and direct patients appropriately.
* Operate the appointment system as directed.
* Extract and file records.
* Regularly repair and tidy records and file letters.
* Answer telephones and take messages.
* Operate the repeat prescription system.
* Keep a day book.
* Record simple statistical information.
* Perform administrative tasks such as registering new patients and filling in forms where directed.
* Serve refreshments.
* Perform other appropriate duties as required.

Every general practitioner who reads this list will want to delete some items and add others. The important point is that each practice should make its own list.

FOR A SECRETARY

A sample description of the duties might be:

* The secretary will receive instructions from and be responsible to the practice manager.
* Open and distribute mail.
* Type letters and documents for the partners and the practice manager.
* Arrange appointments for patients.

* Liaise with hospital secretaries, records departments and admissions office.
* Use age–sex and other registers for arranging follow-up and surveillance of various groups of patients.
* Keep and research information on nursing homes, patients' associations, osteopaths and other agencies which may be of use to patients.
* Maintain diaries for doctors' outside activities.
* Assist in the administration of courses, workshops and other educational activities of the partners.
* Deputise for the practice manager.
* Assist the receptionists if necessary.
* Carry out such other duties as specified by the practice manager.

FOR A PRACTICE MANAGER

A sample description of duties might be:

* The practice manager will receive instructions from and be responsible to the partners.
* Supervise the day-to-day work of the receptionists, secretaries, cleaners and any other non-professional staff.
* Pay staff wages and make the necessary deductions for tax, etc.
* Keep the day-to-day practice accounts in a manner required by the accountants,
* Plan and organise staff training.
* Arrange duty rotas, leave, cover for sick leave, etc.
* Ensure that communications are as effective as possible. Arrange meetings and consultations at all levels.
* Take overall responsibility for the day-to-day running of appointmeent systems, special clinics and other routine activities.
* Ensure that the building is cleaned, maintained and decorated properly.
* Maintain adequate stocks of all medical and non-medical items.
* Liaise with the FPC and make routine returns and claims.
* Keep up to date with NHS regulations.
* Provide support for staff faced with difficult patients.
* Make preliminary investigations into any complaints by patients.
* Liaise with drug company representatives. Arrange and ration interviews.
* Initiate and develop new ideas on practice organisation.

* Audit some aspects of the practice performance.
* Keep statistics of the practice workload.
* Perform such other relevant duties as directed by the partners.

Record-keeping

Record-keeping is the Achilles' heel of many a good practice. Good records are necessary:

* To remind the doctor about previous events and investigations.
* To aid communications in group practices and within the practice team.
* To refer to for medico-legal purposes.
* To use as a teaching aid.
* To implement screening programmes.
* To monitor long-term illnesses.
* To plan continuing care.
* To use as a data base for research.

SIZE OF RECORDS

Most practices use the old Medical Record Envelopes (Lloyd-George MRE), but there has been much discussion about the need to convert GP records to A4 size.

Bigger files should make it easier to store all information and to keep letters, etc. unfolded — but:

1. A big file does not necessarily mean a more orderly or better-kept file (though this should be easier).
2. A small file *might* encourage the doctor to be precise and methodical about recording and to be selective about what is kept.
3. The stationery costs for 3000 A4 records will be in the order of £1000.
4. A4 records need three times as much filing space.

Neat, precise note-keepers will provide excellent small records. Untidy, disorganised people will produce untidy, disorganised A4 records.

FILING SYSTEMS

1. Cabinets
   a. expensive,
   b. take up floor space, but
   c. provide security.
2. Shelving
Lateral filing is easier for retrieval purposes, but
   a. not secure,
   b. needs a lot of wall space.
3. Circular (carousel)
   a. very efficient
   b. Expensive
   c. needs a lot of floor space

Most practices file in alphabetical order. An alternative is to number each record and file them in numerical order — needs a master file to note names and record numbers.

Accurate re-filing is difficult, but can be helped by:

1. Putting a marker in the space the file was taken from.
2. Using the same system but having paired markers — one going into the space and one into the record. This makes it easier to refile quickly.
3. A refinement is to colour-code the markers — revealing who has taken the records out.
4. Tag or colour-code the envelopes to indicate in which drawer or shelf. They are normally filed.

CONTENTS OF THE FILES

The bigger the file and the bigger the jumble of contents, the more irretrievable the information.

* Continuation cards must be in date order.
* Hospital letters and laboratory reports — trimmed to size (use a guillotine) and kept in date order.

* Use treasury tags, staples or flexible pins for keeping notes in order.
* The job of tidying up records must be part of the routine office work. Doctors and staff need regular stimulation to keep notes tidy.
* Unnecessary paper should be discarded. Irrelevant rubbish makes it difficult to get at the importat information — potentially damaging to patient care.
* Most records should be *summarised* — needs a lot of work but worthwhile. Vital if you are going to keep disease registers or become a trainer. Summaries to be typed if possible for doctor to make writing legible. Summarised hospital letters may be thrown away (for some a note may be made of the reference number). Keep anything that may have medico-legal significance (see Figs. 5.4 and 5.5).

RECORDING THE CONSULTATION

Notes must be concise, yet contain relevant important information including important negative findings. Each partnership should evolve its own systems to stimulate some degree of uniformity. It helps retrieval of information if the diagnoses and/or the investigations are boxed or recorded in different-coloured links

AIDING PREVENTION

* Back of envelope only for recording vaccinations.
* Using little labels on front of envelope to jog memory and record BP, smear results, etc.
* Contraception cards with screening reminders.

SPECIAL CARDS

The use of special cards for long-term problems can improve clinical care. The almost universally used example is the antenatal cooperation card. This:

* Collects relevant information together — progress can be followed.

F MALE	SUMMARY OF TREATMENT CARD
Surname SMITH	Forename(s) Eileen
Address 84 Durham Road	
N.H.S. Number	Date of Birth 6/3/41

DATE	CLINICAL NOTES Para 2/0
*1961	PULMONARY TB — (R) apical segmentectomy with PAS/INAH/ Streptomycin for 18 months.
1966	Lassitude/backache — all investigations including Ix NAD c/o Domestic worries. Started on tranquillisers which have continued in variety types/doses ever since. Nervous breakdowns + huge number psych sypts. (E husband homosexual druggaddict → suicide 1967)
1970	Grand mal epilepsy — EEG normal
1975	Asthmatic attacks
1977	2nd husband → Prison (various offences)
1979	Fibroma (L) breast → excised (B)
*1980	Sterilization
1981	Proceedings to ceperate from husband "violence" — dropped
1981	CAT scan normal
1982	Diarrhoea → Ba enema NAD Δ IBS
*	LONG NEUROTIC/HYSTERICAL/SOCIOPATHIC history with frequent psychiatric consultations and admissions. Also sees neurologist re fits *

Dd 8311635 1390M 2/82 A.G. Ltd.   FP9A

Fig. 5.4 Nearly 200 letters were summarised and destroyed. Most were from the patient and her husband to GPs, from GPs to housing and other authorities, from psychiatrists or other hospital consultants to GPs. Forty-seven FP8s were also destroyed — all were for psychiatric/social consultations and multiple psychotropic drug prescriptions. From three large gusseted envelopes this lady's notes were organised into a non-gusseted envelope containing a summary card, a drug card, a current continuation card, thirteen hospital letters and ten representative FP8s.

MALE	SUMMARY OF TREATMENT CARD
Surname WALLACE	Forename(s) William
Address	12 Essex Close
N.H.S. Number	Date of Birth 11/6/49

Date	Clinical Notes
1954	T+A
1961	(R) empyema → decortication (R) lung
1983	Vasectomy

Fig. 5.5 Most patients' notes are easily summarised, and the use of the summary card allows past medical history to be assimilated at a glance.

* Guides clinical care along certain paths.
* Acts as a reminder to do certain regular checks and investigations.

Other special cards can be used for:

Hypertension
Diabetes
Family planning
Epilepsy
Repeat prescribing
Summaries

Examples of these cards are illustrated (Figs. 5.6–5.9). They are not difficult to design and practices could easily produce their own. However, drug companies will provide free cards, particularly for hypertension and contraceptive care and a range of cards are available commercially at very reasonable prices from:

General Practice Supplies
Oakley House
6 Hutton Grove
London N12 8DT

NUTS AND BOLTS

FAMILY PLANNING CARD	DOCTOR Moulds	
Name Ann-Louise GREEN	Date of Birth 15/5/64	Address 4 Kingfishers

PAST HISTORY/RISK FACTORS

PILL	over 35 X	hyperlipidaemia X	jaundice X occasional
	smoker X	hypertension X	migraine ✓ severe tension
	overweight X	diabetes X	CVS disease X headache

COIL/MINI PILL	ectopic pregnancy	OTHERS EPILEPSY
	pelvic inflammation	On Epilim/Phenabarb
	abdominal operations	

GYNAE ASSESSMENT

PARA 0/0	CYCLE 5/21-42	PELVIC EXAM

SCREENING

RUBELLA Vaccinated at school	SMEAR 4/5/83 NAD	BREAST LEAFLET/EXAM

DATE	BP	NOTES	1001 1002
28/x/82	120/60	Wishes pill for contraception. Ovran 50 x 3	1001
14/1/83	BTB at end month. Advised. Ovran 30 x 4 Smear discussed / Risks epilepsy in any children discussed.		
19/4/83	120/60	Well. No fits for few months X 6	
4/5/83		Smear ✓	
4/x/83	120/60	Well X 6	1001

Fig. 5.6 Our family planning card is white and is designed to encourage prevention.

BLOOD PRESSURE CARD							
SURNAME HOLDING				FORENAME Michael			
ADDRESS 24 Westley High Road						D.O.B. 11/6/47	
B.P.		Fundi — I		X Ray			
Wt — Normal || ECG — NAD		Blood FBC	Elect	Lipids	Glucose	VMA.
M.S.U. — NAD || I.V.P.		NAD	NAD			
Comments :- 2/3/83 Routine BP = 190/100 then 210/110 average on 3 occasions.							
Nonsmoker No exercise lean Strong FH	Fundi NAD Femoral pulses normal. Advised re salt / weight / Propranolol 40 mg TID AIM to keep BP at 149/90 or below						

Date	B.P.	Wt.	Urine	Notes
21/4/83	140/100			Propranolol LA male See 1/12
10/5/83	140/100		U/E; FBC; MSU; ECG — all NAD.	
18/5/83	140/95			INDEREX male See 1/12
14/6/83	130/90			Maintain therapy. See 3/12
22/9/83	130/90			See nurse 3/12 See me 6/12

Fig. 5.7a Our blood pressure card is red and used in conjunction with our practice protocol for the management of hypertension, allows us to provide a fairly uniform standard of care.

NAME			DOB	
Initial 1 BPS		2	3	

	RISK FACTORS	
Fam Hist Over wt Smoking	Alcohol Exercise Diabetes	Personality ↑ Lipids

	ASSESSMENT	
Wheezy? Breathless?	Chest pain? Gout?	Cold extremities?

CVS EXAM: FUNDI:		Femoral pulses

	INVESTIGATIONS	
Urine U/E Uric acid	ECG? LFT? IVP??	Lipids?? Glucose?

TRT AIM		

	ADVICE	
Diet/Wt Smoking	Alcohol Exercise	Need for treatment LEAFLET

DATE	BP	NOTES	?Fundi

Fig. 5.7b Our new hypertension card, which we have just introduced to reflect our new protocol, is white with red print. Note how the emphasis has changed from investigations to assessment of risk factors and how much better the new card is at prompting the doctor to find out more about, and communicate better with, the patient.

DIABETES RECORD CARD

Mr./Mrs.	(First Name)		D.O.B.
G.P.	Address		
Date	Initial Assessment		
C.V.S.	B/P		Pulses
C.N.S.	Fundi		Feet

ROUTINE VISITS

- Current Treatment / Other Drugs
- Examination and Comments
- Blood Su: Value, Time
- Urine: Alb, Acet, Sugar
- Wt
- Date

Fig. 5.8 Our diabetes record card is yellow and is meant to be used in conjunction with our protocol. However, unlike our other cards, this one does seem to be too

YEARLY CHECK							
Date	C.V.S.	B/P	C.N.S.	Pulses	Fundi	Feet	

ROUTINE VISITS

	Current Treatment Other Drugs									
	Examination and Comments									
	Blood Su	Value								
		Time								
	Urine	Alb								
		Acet								
		Sugar								
	Wt									
	Date									

much like hard work to keep up to date. As we are tending to avoid using it, we will soon have to decide whether to make another effort or to scrap it and redesign something simpler.

Epilepsy Card				
SURNAME		FORENAMES	D of B	SEX
DATE OF FIRST FIT				
TYPE OF FITS				
AETIOLOGY				
CONFIRMED BY E.E.G.				
CONSULTANT				
PLAN				
REVIEW EVERY				
FBC and RED CELL FOLATE EVERY				
SERUM Ca. P. and ALK. PHOS. EVERY				
OCCUPATION				

COUNSELLING CHECK LIST

TABLET TAKING		AVOIDANCE OF PRECIPITATING FACTORS	
FREE PRESCRIPTION		WHAT TO DO FOR A FIT	
DRIVING		FEARS FOR FUTURE	
MEDIC ALERT		GENETIC	
BRITISH EPILEPSY ASSN.		LITERATURE	
WATER and HEIGHTS			

Fig. 5.9 This is the only commercially designed card that we use. As it fitted

DATE	FREQUENCY OF FITS	SIDE EFFECTS	TREATMENT	SERUM LEVEL	Hb.	RED CELL FOLATE	Ca.	P.	ALK. PHOS.

© 1980 GPS., FREEPOST, BUSHEY, WATFORD, WD2 1FP GPS 7

with our own epilepsy protocol, we bought a quantity from General Practice Supplies.

The age–sex register

An age-sex register is a data retrieval system. When working properly, regularly updated and fully utilised it should improve patient care, increase practice income, and have the potential to act as a research tool.

It separates the practice population into males and females, groups them chronologically according to year of birth and arranges them alphabetically within their year group.

The simplest system is a manual card index — blue cards for males and pink for females. The most basic information would be name, address date of birth. To this could be added marital status, social status, and the date they joined the practice (see Fig. 5.10) and then details about immunisation, family planning or cervical cytology. It could also incorporate a disease code or a record of patients on regular therapy.

At first sight the RCGP cards look daunting, but have all these options. Each card when filled in is placed on a tray with others of the same 'year of birth', separated by marker boards from preceding or subsequent years, the whole being contained in a cabinet.

The information available can be demonstrated by going to each year marker, e.g. in 1983 going to the marker for:

1948 Identifies all those women who are 35.
Do they need contacting for cervical cytology?
1967 Probable school-leavers.
Time for a tetanus toxoid and polio booster?
1973 Identifies 10-year-old girls who could be sent a birthday card — offering rubella vaccination plus a free gift (the latter could be worth about 50p — a tax deductible expense — offset against item-of-service fee) — to encourage attendance for immunisation and help achieve a practice rate of 100 per cent.

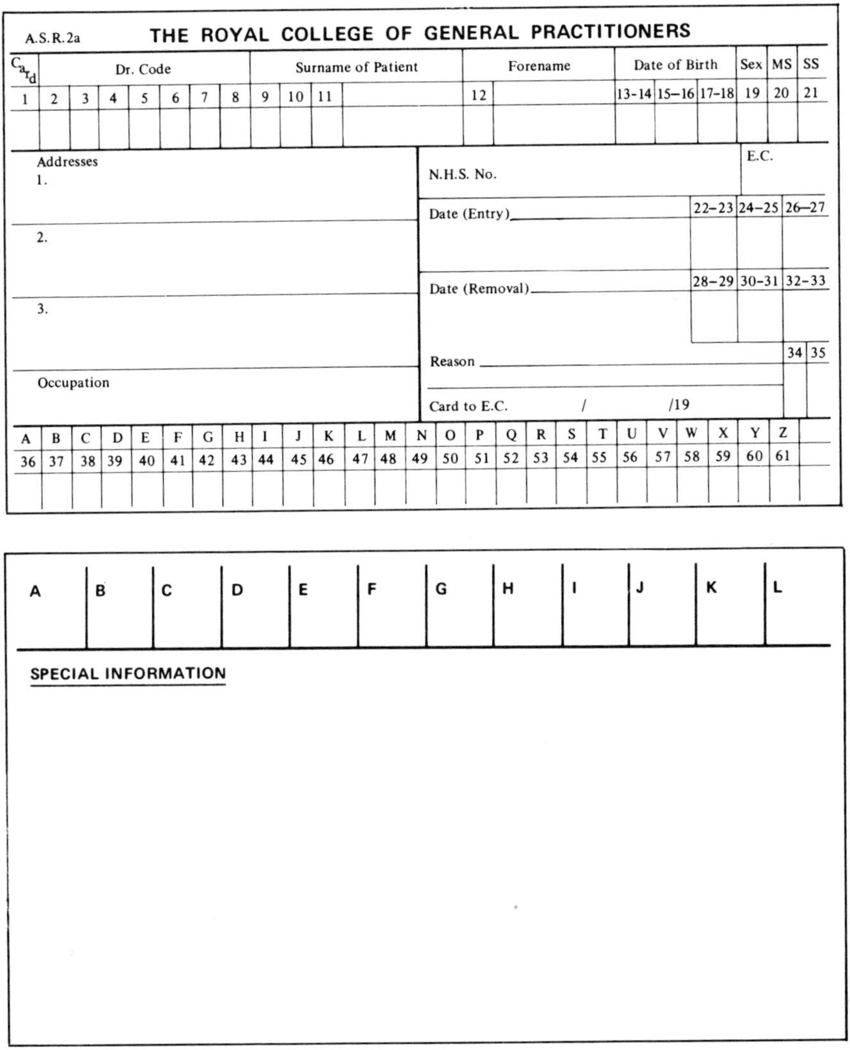

Fig. 5.10 The RCGP age–sex register card

1978 Preschool children — in need of booster for tetanus toxoid and polio?
1981 Have they all had their measles and triple?

At the other end of the scale identify the over-65s (1918) and the 75s (1908). Does the practice feel they should be seen by someone from the team each year?

Having set up an excellent system, the most difficult part is yet to come. Somebody must be delegated to ensure it is maintained accurately and that it is up to date. Like painting the Forth Bridge, this is a never-ending task.

Immunisation systems

FOR CHILDREN

Everyone connected with the practices' immunisation programme should speak with one voice. Practitioners should:

* confidently promote the benefits of immunisation
* advise strongly that immunisation is desirable
* recommend immunisation whenever possible
* discuss the pros and cons whenever asked to
* possess a sound knowledge, particularly of contra-indications

A practice policy allows everyone to give consistent advice. If one partner becomes the practice vaccination authority, then he or she can take the responsibility for sorting out parents' worries. The practice nurses and health visitors should be actively involved.

FOLLOW-UP BABIES

1. Make out card (Fig. 5.11) or fill in birth book (Fig. 5.12) for every baby born into or joining the practice. Health visitors, clerks or receptionists can do this job.
2. At the end of each month all completed cards are put in a box file in the nurses' treatment room. There they are indexed by month of birth and filled in by nurse after she has carried out any vaccination and sent off the form claiming payment.
3. At the end of each month one of the health visitors extracts the cards from the months where babies would be at least one month overdue for any of the main vaccinations and checks them — e.g. at end of May 1984 she looks through the cards of babies filed

```
ANDREW  JONES    DOB  15/7/81     Dr. Martin
80 Northey

1. (DPT)/ DT /(Polio)         ✓ 20/10/82
2. (DPT)/ DT /(Polio)         ✓ 16/12/82
3.  DPT/ DT/  Polio
4.  Measles.
```

Fig. 5.11 A card for each baby filed by month of birth allows an easy check on overdue vaccinations

January 1983

Date	Name	6/52	Immunisations	7½	14/12	Measles	2yr	3½	4½	Pre-school booster

Fig. 5.12 The 'birth book' allows for rapid identification of non-attenders for immunisation, and for smaller practices is probably more useful than the card index system

under the months of birth January 1984 — should have had first triple and polio; November 1983 — should have had second triple and polio; May 1983 — should have had third triple and polio; November 1982 — should have had measles.

Any baby she finds that is not fully vaccinated to date is visited until either vaccination is effected or the card annotated to say that the parents have consciously refused vaccination. (The birth book can be used in the same way and is probably more useful for small practices, while the card index system is better if a lot of babies need following up.)

4. While this is going on the doctor can help by quickly scanning the back of the record envelope, reserved solely for recording im-

munisations or natural measles infection, at any consultation with children and so can identify gaps. Advice to parents there and then can motivate them to protect their child.
5. One doctor audits every six months to determine the practice rates which, if low, show where improvement is needed or, if high, allow praise to be lavished on all concerned, so encouraging them to do even better in the future.

Using the card index system our audit for babies born in the six months from March–August 1981 inclusive showed that: out of a total of 186 babies, 8 left the practice before or during their vaccination course. Of the 178 still with us:

97.2% were covered against DT and polio (80% nationally)
82% were covered against pertussis (less than 50% nationally)
64% were covered against measles (50% nationally)

FOR TRAVELLERS

The protective measures recommended will depend on the countries to be visited, the length of stay and the conditions under which the traveller is expected to live. There are too many variables involved to feel confident that a practice nurse will have the necessary breadth of knowledge to take account of them all.

To ensure comprehensive and up-to-date advice, one or two partners should be responsible for providing this aspect of care to all the practice patients.

1. Patient requests advice or vaccinations for travel.
2. Is given form (Fig. 5.13) to fill in by reception staff, nurses or doctor. Asked to see nurse in two days re vaccination.
3. Filled-in form is passed to doctor, who makes out vaccination plan (after referring to *Pulse's Foreign Travel Guide* and patient's current status), malaria prophylaxis and instructions for nurse.
4. Fully completed form goes to practice nurse, who discusses plan with patient. Plan used to record vaccination given. Nurse fills in FP73' and appropriate certificates. Nurse gives patient copy of DHSS leaflet SA35 'Protect your health abroad'
5. Certificates and FP73s to doctor for completion. Doctor writes out prescription for vaccines bought by practice (at end of month all prescriptions sent to the FPC on form FP34 to get cost of vaccine plus prescription payments; NB: This applies to non-

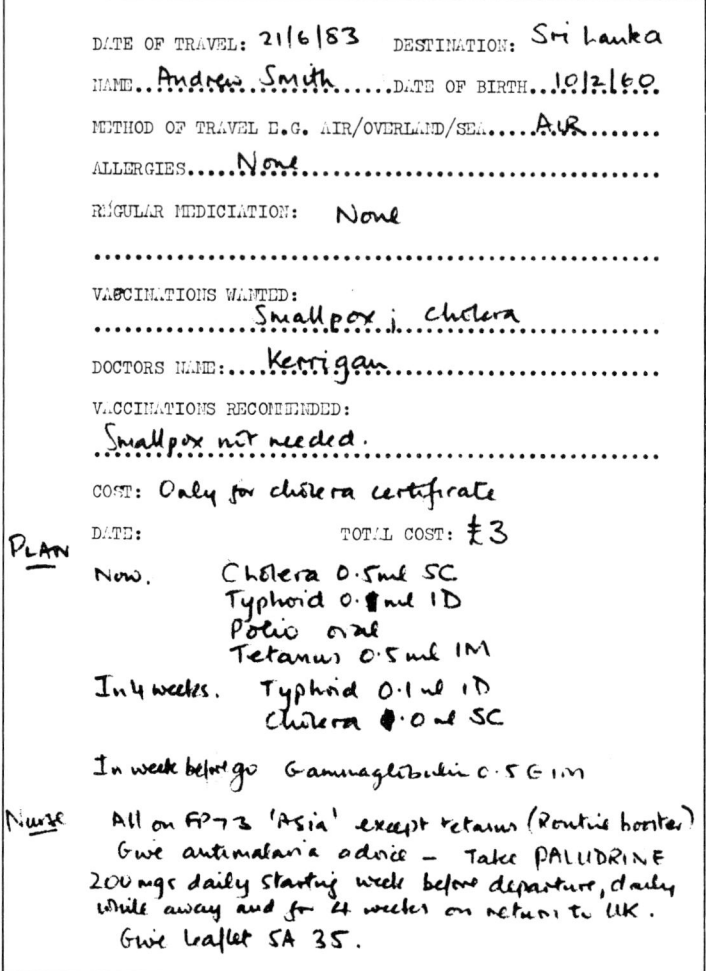

Fig. 5.13 Practice travel form.

dispensing doctors) and private prescription for anti-malaria tablets if required.
6. At end of vaccination course patient pays reception staff and collects appropriate certificates and prescriptions.

Repeat prescribing systems

Up to 50 per cent of all prescriptions issued are repeats for patients on regular medication. Last year our practice issued over 27 000. Each doctor does about thirteen repeat prescriptions each working day.

In view of the importance of this activity, an efficient system to allow for the easy, accurate, appropriate, economical and carefully monitored provision of these items should be devised.

Such a system should not be used to keep patients away from the doctor for long periods of time, but should be used to monitor patients with chronic conditions and to ensure that those patients who have not been seen for a reasonable length of time can be asked to reattend.

Although much of the administrative work can be carried out by practice staff, their role should be confined to administration and should not include any responsibilty for writing out the actual drugs or dosages being prescribed.

This work can be computerised to decrease doctor prescribing workload, while strengthening controls over prescribing and increasing the effectiveness of follow-up patients on long-term medication.

ORGANISATION OF A SYSTEM

1. When patient is on regular medication doctor fills in repeat drug card (Fig. 5.14) which is inserted in the record envelope. At same time fills in patient's repeat card (Fig. 5.15) to show when card is valid to.
2. When a patient wants a repeat prescription, the card is handed in to reception. The receptionist logs the request in a large loose-leaf

REPEAT PRESCRIPTIONS		
Surname	Forename(s)	
Relevant Conditions		Card Issued
DRUGS		
Date	Name, Strength and Dose	Number
	NEXT DATE TO BE SEEN	

Fig. 5.14 Our repeat prescription cards are bright yellow and can be easily identified in the notes.

repeat prescription request folder and fills in an FP10 with the patient's name and address. If the card is no longer valid or if any items have been requested which are not on the current treatment regimen, then the receptionist gets the patient's medical record envelope out.

DATE	DRUGS	DATE	DRUGS	DATE	DRUGS

3. All cards/envelopes are collected in a box, and each day the box and the request folder are taken to the common room to be "processed" by the doctors at the end of morning surgery.
4. If a card is no longer valid, the patient's notes are scrutinised to see whether the patient should be requested to come for follow-

				LAINDON HEALTH CENTRE
THIS CARD IS VALID UNTIL				REPEAT PRESCRIPTION CARD

Surname _____ Forename(s) _____

Address _____

Doctor _____

AFTER THE LATEST DATE SHOWN ABOVE YOUR TREATMENT MUST BE REVIEWED BY THE DOCTOR
PLEASE REMEMBER TO ALLOW AT LEAST 24 HOURS FOR US TO PROCESS YOUR PRESCRIPTION MONDAY TO FRIDAY OR
48 HOURS AT WEEKENDS   LHC 18

To get a repeat prescription you should put this card in the special box in the health centre
Prescriptions will usually be ready for collection 24 hours later.
Please DO NOT USE THE TELEPHONE unless there is an emergency.
A stamped addressed envelope should be supplied if you want the prescription posted to you.
This card is only valid until the date shown on the back.

CURRENT TREATMENT

	DRUGS, STRENGTH, DOSE	No:	DATE	DRUGS	DATE	DRUGS
1						
2						
3						
4						
5						
6						
7						
8						
9						
10						

Fig. 5.15 The repeat prescription card helps patients, receptionists and doctors to gain an accurate prescription with the minimum of bother. It also allows the doctor to retain control over the patient's drug-taking habits and to ensure appropriate follow-up.

up. If so, a standard note is attached to the card, if not, the 'valid until' box is amended and a prescription issued.

5. All completed prescriptions — ticked off in the request folder — are taken back to reception and issued to patients or relatives as they request them.

Computers

Computers are non-intelligent machines that can store, recall and analyse data rapidly. They are worthy of consideration in any practice that is anxious to improve data storage and analysis, repreat prescribing and screening and preventative programmes.

FUNCTIONS OF GP SYSTEMS

Computer systems now on offer can perform most of the following functions — with varying degrees of efficiency:

Age–sex register   Normally with space to record ten to twenty-other items of information such as address, NHS number, social class, etc. Capacity varies from system to system

Morbidity registers, disease registers   Capacity varies a lot. Very limited if entered in free text. Most need the operator to code the disease first — which is laborious. One or two systems only will actually do the coding for you. Search and analysis facilities — vital if you want to do research. Vary a lot.

Recall registers   Facility to recall patients for review or for screening purposes, though with no guarantee they will attend!

Repeat prescribing   The only function that *really* saves work for the doctor and staff. Some have drug interactions warning systems. Only one has a complete drug dictionary in the memory.

Accounting   Many commercial programmes are available.

Word processing   programmes are available with most systems. Useful for routine letters, particularly if used with the recall system.

Search and analysis facilities   Some systems offer very little. More powerful systems allow you to search all the files and to analyse the data in almost any way you wish.

Records   Only the biggest and most powerful systems are suitable for routine record-keeping.

THE SNAGS

Many GPs have unrealistic expectations of computer systems and must be careful to assess all the implications in terms of money and work.

Monday   Quoted prices are often without VAT. Allocate 10–15 per cent of the purchase price per annum for maintenance insurance.

Work   The work involved in putting even the most basic data into the system is *enormous*. Most practices take at least a year to do this. If any disease registers are kept, the doctors will have to do a lot of work labelling and summarising notes.

Staffing   Reception staff are often wary of new technology. You will need extra staff.

Rewards   Satisfaction only — do not believe sales pitches that imply that extra fees generated will pay for the system.

WHICH SYSTEM TO CHOOSE

Make sure you know exactly what you want the computer to do for you.

Give suppliers a written specification and make sure that the system quoted will do everything you want.

A good system will:

* make data input *easy*
* enable staff to become computer-proficient quickly
* not be tiring to use
* have a big enough memory
* be expandable
* preferably be capable of being used by more than one person at a time
* be able to code and search all data

Suppliers should be able to give a reasonable guarantee and long-term back-up for the hardware and the software.

Patient education

Patient education should form a large part of any consultation. It is often said that the word 'doctor' means 'teacher' and not 'treater', and it is in this role that GPs are probably most effective whether they are discussing the self-limiting course of childhood illnesses, the dangers of failure to have infants immunised, or the need to take life-long therapy in a case of hypertension.

The education in a consultation can be reinforced in many ways. First of all, every member of the primary care team should speak with one voice and give consistent replies to many of the common questions patients ask. Nothing is more disruptive for a young mother with her first child than to be given conflicting advice on how to manage nappy rash. Even worse, of course, is the minefield of infant feeding.

Thus the health visitor, the midwives and the treatment room nurses should try to develop some common ideas. In the waiting room this may be reinforced with slide projector carousels offering health education advice by flashing a message onto a screen.

During a consultation, why not give a booklist, or offer the address of a self-help group? Reading or socialising may drive home a point far more clearly than the doctor's phrases; after all, the average patient can only remember three things in any one consultation.

Why not offer suitable patients a leaflet about their condition? Those points you wish to get over are more properly learnt in the less frenetic atmosphere outside the surgery, and time is saved in the consultation itself. Further advantages are that there is now a guarantee that the patient has all the relevant information (there is no guarantee that the doctor will remember to transmit all the essentials orally), and relatives and friends can also learn about the patient's problem (rather than pick up garbled, misheard information).

There are many sources for good leaflets, and all should be taken advantage of: The Health Education Council 'self-help groups' summaries from articles in books and magazines — both medical and lay' and drug companies. The *Patient Counselling Compendium* available from PCA Ltd, Marlborough, Wiltshire SN8 IBR is especially useful for advice sheets on common problems such as piles, varicose veins and hay fever. When there is no source to crib from, then self-help is the answer.

HOW TO PREPARE A PATIENT INFORMATION LEAFLET

Aims

* To reinforce what the doctor has said.
* A source to which the patient can refer either now or in the future.
* To encourage the patient to be self-reliant.

Message

* An indication of the severity and frequency of the problem.
* Equate risk factors with everyday parameters, e.g. the risk of death on the roads.
* Point out side-effects, forestall patient's objections and foresee difficulties that may occur.
* When to seek further medical help.

Style

* Should be *Daily Mirror*, not *Daily Telegraph*.
* Anglo-Saxon not Latin word-roots — but not patronising.
* Crisp, clear, direct phrases — little equivocation.
* Short sentences — mixture of upper and lower case. Remember capitals, thick print, directions in boxes are a turn-off.

Layout

* Short paragraphs.
* Adopt the style "But what if I have..." and give the answer.
* Notice how *Readers Digest* address their letters personally. Leave space for the personal touch — the autograph and the talisman.

Audit

* When you next see the patient, ask how helpful the leaflet was.
* Prepare a small questionnaire on its value.
* Ask direct questions — the answers to which should be in the text.

The leaflet below on warts is one that we wrote and use.

WARTS AND VERRUCAS

Warts are caused by a virus and affect up to 10 per cent of the population at any one given time. They are infectious, and spread by contact during hand-holding games and from walking barefoot on gymasium or swimming-pool floors. The large majority of cases occur in children, and in most of them the wart will disappear by itself within a few months. This is because the child develops immunity and kills the virus off. At the outside, this process will take 2–3 years, and afterwards no more warts will be caught.

A verruca is a wart which happens to be on the foot. Unlike other warts, it may be painful and it can become pressed into the soles of the feet by the pressure of walking.

Before any treatment for a wart is undertaken, *consider:*

1. Warts go away by themselves in children.
2. There is no drug effective against the wart virus.
3. Most treatments have poorer results than leaving the wart alone.
4. Treatment is often painful, while the wart is usually painless.
5. A wart going away by itself leaves no scars, while treatment may do.
6. If a wart is removed before the patient has got immunity, then he will catch the next wart he comes into contact with.

Unless a wart/verruca is painful or producing an unacceptable deformity:

NO TREATMENT IS NEEDED

Where you wish to treat a wart — covering it daily with a waterproof plaster for 6–8 weeks may well destroy it.

Where you wish to treat a verruca, the following treatment is often effective.

1. Emery board or nail file removal of dry skin around verruca.
2. Soak verruca and surrounding area in a saucer containing 5 per

cent formalin solution (can be obtained at chemist) for 15 minutes.
3. If formalin will go near or on the toes, then protect them by smearing them with Vaseline before soaking.
4. Rinse the formalin, repeating the treatment daily for six weeks.

IF A WART/VERRUCA IS CAUSING PROBLEMS OR IS RESISTANT TO TREATMENT, THEN CONSULT YOUR DOCTOR.

Preparing a practice protocol

Clinical freedom is regarded by many doctors as a divine right. This 'right' should not extend to being allowed to practise in sloppy, illogical, bad or even dangerous ways.

A partnership, or other group of interested doctors, should be able to sit down together to reach a consensus view on what would constitute reasonable and desirable standards of care for a given condition. Once such a protocol has been devised, while it cannot be rigidly adhered to all the time every time, it should not be deviated from without an identifiable and logical reason.

The preparation of a practice protocol should go through the following phases:

1. Partners define which areas of practice would benefit from a unified approach, e.g. antenatal care, management of hypertension, follow-up of epileptics, diabetic care, contraceptive care.
2. A partner is nominated to research the subject and to prepare a discussion document with recommendations.
3. Discussion document circulated to all partners for comment.
4. A time is set for a discussion or series of discussions with the objective of reaching a consensus opinion. NB: this implies a willingness among all concerned to change behaviour which is not based on clear-cut factual evidence.
5. A programme for implementation is devised.
6. After 6–12 months an audit is carried out to test the effectiveness of, and adherence to the standards set by, the protocol.

Our antenatal protocol is one among many which has been arrived at in this way. Simple as it is, some of us still experience difficulties in departing from the habits of a clinical lifetime to follow its recommendations.

ANTENATAL PROTOCOL

Diagnosis

Clinical whenever possible. Gravindex only if diagnosis is in doubt or if chemical confirmation of pregnancy is necessary, e.g. pre TOP.

Booking

Patient to book at reception for practice antenatal clinic coinciding with 10–12 weeks' gestation.
Receptionist to raise form FP 24 with booking date and patient's signature.
Give bottle for urine sample for first attendance.

First antenatal attendance

Reception: Raise practice antenatal and cooperation cards, form FW8 and tag record envelope for antenatal care.
Clinic: Test and record urine and weight.
Midwife/health visitor: Long interview to discuss

* aims of antenatal care
* healthy diet
* breastfeeding/breast care
* smoking
* any problem the patient wishes to bring up
* mothercraft/relaxation classes
* give leaflets/booklets on healthy pregnancy, etc.

Doctor (NB: if patient does not request a particular doctor try to put in with registered doctor): Fill in antenatal and cooperation cards noting relevant social, medical and obstetric history. Check teeth, examine abdomen, listen to heart, examine breasts. Do BP.
Advise patient re booking procedure for hospital element of antenatal care. Make date for next practice appointment. Give opportunity to discuss any other problems or worries.
NB: no home or GP unit deliveries, Discuss pros/cons with any patient wishing a home delivery and advise that she need only be in hospital for 8–12 hours for delivery and we will look after her at home the rest of the time.

Subsequent examinations

At 20, 26, 30, 34, 36 weeks, then weekly.
If patient attends hospital antenatal clinic, then she should not attend us in the same week.
Reception: Welcome patient and ask which doctor she wishes to see.
Clinic: Check urine and weight. Answer any problems or queries the patient may bring up.
Doctor: Check fundus, BP, ankles for oedemna. Ask re any problems or worries. Enter and note details of blood group, rubella status, rhesus antibody status and haemoglobin on cards as results become available. Check initial MSU result.
Haemoglobin — to be done at first hospital booking then at 28 weeks (give form at 26 week attendance) and 32 weeks.
Rh antibodies — as requested by lab. Normally booking, 26, 32, 36 weeks and term.
Iron — at 20 week attendance check result of booking Hb. If < 12G; PH iron deficiency or poor social/dietary background prescribe cheapest iron/folate preparation (Folex 350) and ensure patient understands why it must be taken regularly.
Other women should be advised they have no need to take iron unless they really wish to but that their blood will be rechecked at 28 weeks to ensure that they are still all right. No unthinking prescription of iron.

POSTNATAL CARE

If patient discharged in 48 hours or less then 2 postnatal visits by doctor. Otherwise only 1 routine visit.

At visit

Check on breasts, abdomen, perineum. Examine baby and ask about feeding. Ask about contraceptive intentions. Remind mother about baby clinic and inoculations. Rubella vaccination for seronegative women. Review iron therapy and BP is indicated.

Postnatal examination

This should take place between 7–12 weeks.

Check weight, BP, Hb if appropriate. Pelvic examination if patient wishes or if patient has not resumed satisfactory sexual intercourse. Advise re contraception. Fill in FP 1001.

Complete antenatal card, then discard all unnecessary hospital letters and lab reports relating to the pregnancy. Complete FP24 and attach to front of record envelope for action by reception staff.

Practical audit

Gathering information about a variety of practice activities allows constructive analysis to see exactly what is happening rather than what everyone either thinks, or hopes, is going on. Work done is analysed regularly, though not necessarily frequently, so allowing practice responses to be devised to deal with problems uncovered. All partners take part, and any partner can look into any aspect of practice activity that is of interest. The others may help in the gathering of specific information, but usually only become really involved when the results are presented and discussed.

Self and practice audit carried out in a cooperative and friendly spirit is stimulating, exciting and good fun. It also improves the standard of care given to practice patients.

BACKGROUND INFORMATION

To put our audit results in perspective, it helps to know a little about the practice:

It has nine doctors: seven full-time males, two half-time females.

There are 23 500 patients: 10 per cent over 65 (16 per cent nationally). Social bias heavily to classes 3, 4 and 5.

We have five practice nurses and two nurse practitioners. They effect nearly one in three of all patient/practice consultations and carry out one in three of our in-hours home visits. They run smear and family planning clinics and carry out a wide range of paramedical as well as nursing duties.

The annual doctor/patient consultation rate is 2.35/patient.

The annual doctor home visiting rate (in hours) is 0.2/patient.

The annual doctor home visiting rate (out of hours) is 0.08/patient.

Total patient/doctor interactions are 2.6/patient/year. NB: this is well below average, but once the nurse/patient interaction of one per patient per year is added in, a total patient/medical interaction rate of 3.6 is reached. This is about average for the doctor/patient rates nationally. ("Out of hours" is defined as between 6 p.m. and 9 a.m.)

AUDIT

Some of the recent audits that we have undertaken are discussed below. None of them took more than a few hours to do, and similiar exercises could be usefully carried out by any reasonably cohesive partnership.

1. Question

As our patients can see any doctor, how many actually see the doctor they are registered with?

Audit A simple check of 200 consecutive consultations for each doctor showed that 74 per cent of patients were seeing their own doctor; 20 per cent a doctor in the group of four their doctor worked in; and only 6 per cent a doctor in the other group.

Conclusion Our patients do not move about as much as we thought they did, and more than seven out of ten of them choose to see their own doctor. NB: we also surveyed our patients to find that 50 per cent of them wanted, as far as possible, always to see 'their' doctor, while the other 50 per cent wanted to be free to consult any doctor.

2. Question

Do we see the same type of problems/patients and treat them in the same way?

Audit A simple form was devised (Fig. 5.16) to allow each partner to record information about 200 consecutive consultations. Noted for each consultation was the patient's age, sex, diagnostic group (S = skins, P = psychiatric, G = gynae, etc.), accute or chronic conditions, doctor or patient-initiated consultation, and type of prescriptions given, if any.

Easy addition allowed each doctor to arrive at percentage figures showing what proportions of his or her consultations were with females, with different age — groups, in broad diagnostic groups,

No.	Age	Sex	Acute (A) Chronic (C)	Patient or doctor initiated	Diagnostic group	Prescription or not
1	24	♀	A	P	G	Canestan
2	5	♂	A	P	R	Advice
3	42	♀	A	P	R	Advice
4						
5						
6						
7						
8						
9						
10						
11						
12						
13						
14						
15						
16						
17						
18						
19						
20						

Acute = A Patient initiated = P Diagnostic groups: S = Skins
Chronic = C Doctor initiated = D   E = Emotional
                                                      M = Musculoskeletal
                                                      R = Respiratory
                                                      Gy = Gynae
                                                      GI = Gastrointestinal
                                                      O = Other

Fig. 5.16 A simple system of recording can be easily devised to suit any practice's needs.

for acute conditions, recalled, and prescribed for, and if so what was prescribed.

An entertaining evening was had by all discussing the results. These showed some, already suspected, differences in age/sex distribution of patients seen but, more significantly, that one partner had a very high recall rate and a very high prescribing rate for children, and that one other had a far higher prescribing rate than our average.

Conclusion With two exceptions we were all seeing broadly the same problems without too great a disparity in our recall or prescribing rates.

3. Question

Although our practice prescribing costs are less than half the national average, are they in fact hiding significant variations in the prescribing habits of individual partners?

Audit As our policy is to advise rather than to prescribe for self-limiting conditions, one partner decided to look at prescribing for minor ailments. To do this he kept looking through records until he had recorded the outcome of 100 'minor' consultations for each doctor. The consultations were all taken from 1981–82 and were all for problems where there was an obvious choice about whether a prescription should be given or not, e.g. colds, coughs, flu, sore throats, catarrh, earache, diarrhoea, vomiting, colic warts, verrucas, non-specific rashes, insomnia, being 'run down', anxiety, aches/pains, injuries and dysuria.

The figures showed that a range from 25–69 per cent of these kind of patients were given prescriptions. Of even more interest was the finding that the average for the four trainers in the practice was 28 per cent, while for the non-trainers it was 55 per cent. For a composite 100 consultations from three trainees, their average was 38 per cent. We also found that most of us had specific prescribing 'problems'. The highest prescriber was let down by his inability not to prescribe penicillin for virtually every URTI (despite it being our policy not to do so), while one of the lowest prescribers would have been lower still if he hadn't prescribed for every backache he saw, whatever its severity.

Conclusion Our non-trainers prescribe as well as advising, while our trainers are much better at saying 'no'. In fact, if our two most reflex prescribers were not included, the other seven partners' average was 36 per cent.

Our non-prescribing policy is working over the practice as a whole, but two partners might think more before automatically reaching for FP10s.

A reaudit next year will show whether there has been any change in habits.

4. Question

As a practice and as individuals, what do we refer to hospital outpatients?

Audit One partner felt she might be referring a higher proportion of patients to hospital than the rest of us. She got the secretaries to tabulate a six-month block of referrals by doctor and by specialty referred to. The results showed that among us we referred 1089 patients to outpatients in a six-month period and that a significant majority of these referrals were for surgical intervention of one form or another. Only 31 were to psychiatrists and 83 to physicians (remembering also that many of these were for those X-ray examinations we cannot get done directly).

Individual doctors were shown to have broadly the same referral rates overall, but there were also some marked differences in referral rates to individual specialities. We are now getting all the notes out for those patients referred by the highest referring partner for each speciality. Each referral will be discussed to see if it was legitimate or whether it could have been better dealt with in a different way.

Conclusion As 15 per cent of the population are new referrals to outpatients each year, we seem to be coping pretty well with our workload, only needing to refer about 9 per cent of our patients annually to hospital.

5. Question

Is our hypertension screening programme working?

Audit For three years now we have been trying to do BPs in all 35–65-year-olds. One partner took a random 200 records of patients in this age group and counted the number that had had their BP taken. Seventy-two per cent of them had, many of the remainder had not attended for three years, though a distinct minority had attended many times without having a BP taken. This interesting sub-group were easily recognised by us as patients either whose departure from the surgery we did not wish to delay, even for the few seconds needed to take a BP, or as patients in whom there was so much else going on that no-one wanted to find anything else!

Conclusion Our programme is working, but we must keep up the effort. A similar audit for our cervical cytology programme showed that 75 per cent of our 20–60-year-old female patients had had a smear within the past five years.

6. Question

Does our policy of providing a comprehensive, up-to-date family planning service for our patients pay off?

Audit In 1982 we had 1650 FP 1001s and 146 FP 1002s signed. This figure has increased every year for many years and is considerably in excess of the average 100 FP 1001s per GP per annum in the country as a whole — even after taking into account our larger list sizes.

Conclusion For 1982 the practice earned £15,600 from our contraceptive service — a well worthwhile return for our enthusiastic approach and our rubella, smear and breast self-examination programmes.

7. Question

How good are we at putting in coils?

Audit Five partners put in about 150 coils among them each year. Virtually all are copper 7s and are put in at ordinary surgery appointments. One partner, who puts in the most, wanted to repeat an audit of 500 coils (1000 years of coil use) that we did a few years ago, so he got one of the secretaries to abstract the notes of 100 patients from our coil register.

Analysis of 200 years of coil use — total insertions 100, 97 ours, 3 from hospital showed:

4 coils removed due to menorrhagia/dysmenorrhoea
2 accidental pregnancies
1 definite and 1(?) salpingitis
8 expulsions
0 perforations

The definite salpingitis and two of the expulsions were in the three coils that had been inserted at the hospital, so our figures are in fact better than shown.

Conclusion Our rates for coil complications are as good, if not better, than those generally reported. This is most reassuring, as we are continually being told by the experts that GPs often do not put in enough coils to maintain insertion skills.

The results are the same as we found with our previous 500 coil audit.

Our audit information is now kept in a folder and can be referred to by any partner. Keeping the results makes for interesting comparisons in the future.

Learning about the consultation

This section is intended to provide a framework for learning about the consultation. It is difficult to change an established pattern of behaviour, so it is not surprising that general practitioners after adopting a particular style of consultation do not vary it to any great extent. The researches of Byrne and Long showed that the majority of general practitioners used the same techniques irrespective of the nature of the problem being presented by the patient.

The young doctor is trained to conduct a consultation on a question-and-answer basis. The interrogation leads to a physical examination, followed by the formulation of a diagnosis. The doctor in his or her wisdom then gives directive advice and treatment. This model is appropriate when there is straightforward physical illness, but even here the intelligent adult may wish to have adequate explanation and to be involved in any decision-making. For the patient with emotional or social problems, a non-directive style is more likely to allow the expression of feelings and emotions and the generation of self-solutions to the problems.

You have only to ask yourself: Do you employ a range of consultation techniques and do you use them appropriately?

The best way to find out about your own behaviour is to make tape, or better still, video recordings of consultations.

ANALYSIS OF THE RECORDINGS

These are best done:

* First by the doctor who made the recording. This allows him or her to identify strengths and weaknesses and to think about what happened, before showing it to others.

* Subsequently, in a small group with colleagues who are friendly and are capable of being supportive:
    1. The doctor gives his or her own views first.
    2. The group must praise the good points before offering constructive criticism.

LOOKING AT CONSULTATIONS

Before attempting to analyse recordings, it is important to have a theoretical framework of the consultation from which to work. Break up the consultation into its various phases and examine how the conduct of the consultation proceeded, and if the necessary tasks were achieved. The structure that follows is useful but by no means comprehensive, and you may well wish to construct your own.

The greeting

  * Is it appropriate? Does it establish rapport?
  * Look for eye contact and vocal and facial expressions.

Defining the problem

  * Why did the patient come to the surgery today? Look at the way the doctor obtains information from the patient.
  * What kind of questions are asked? Closed questions, e.g. 'Are you depressed?' This only allows a yes or no answer. Open question, e.g. 'How do you feel about the situation?' This allows the patient the opportunity to control the direction of the consultation.
  * Note whether the doctor allows the patient time to think, uses silence to give the initiative to the patient or uses encouraging noises to make the patient feel he or she has the doctor's attention.
  * Body language is important. Does the doctor look interested and accessible?
  * Finally, was the task of finding out why the patient came achieved? Judgment is often subjective and is particularly difficult if the method of interrogation is inappropriate.

The physical examination

  * Was it skilful? Was it appropriate?

Exploring the patient's ideas

* Has the patient been encouraged to express his or her own ideas about the nature and management of the problem?

Finding solutions

* Was the process used for identifying a solution appropriate to the patient and was the outcome reasonable?
* The doctor gives advice — appropriate for the clear-cut organic problem needing action — "You have appendicitis and you will have to go into hospital".
* The doctor provides two or three possible alternative solutions and then discusses the pros and cons with the patient, e.g. offers the Pill and the coil as possible methods of contraception for the women who has just had a baby.
* The doctor avoids giving advice. Helps the patient to formulate his or her own solutions to the problem. This "counselling" approach is non-directive and is appropriate for the patient who has social and emotional problems.

The use of time and terminating the consultation

* Were the overall strategies employed by the doctor suitable for a routine general practice consultation?
* Look at the use of time and the use of resources.
     Was the consultation terminated kindly and efficiently?

Recording consultations

* Talk to your vocational training course organiser. He or she should have considerable experience in these methods.
* Borrow a recorder from the course or ask your regional GP adviser.
* Make sure your patients are informed that they are being recorded.
* Set up a group of colleagues who will look at the results. If you find this difficult, the local trainers workshop will almost certainly be able to help.

For further information read Byrne and Long, *Doctors Talking to Patients*, HMSO and Pendleton et al *The Consultation — An Approach to Learning and Teaching* Oxford University Press.

Becoming a training practice

Benefits

A practice will benefit in many ways from training:

Mental stimulation The presence of a trainee with an enquiring mind banishes complacency and makes the partners think about what they are doing.

Improving practice standards Teaching practices will be expected to have above-average standards. The competition and the rationalisation of work will eventually provide the patients with better and more appropriate care.

Improving the overall standards of GPs The GPs of today have a duty to provide the best possible training for their successors. Good training must eventually lead to better overall standards.

Improving practice income The trainers' grant and extra fees from lecturing and other teaching activities make a substantial addition to practice income.

WHAT IS REQUIRED OF A TEACHING PRACTICE

The criteria for the selection of trainers are becoming ever more stringent.

Motivation to teach The prospective trainer must demonstrate that he or she wants to teach and enjoys teaching. Evidence of other teaching activities will help to convince the selectors.

Ability to teach The trainer will have to be willing to learn the theory and skills of teaching. This means attendance at trainer's courses and workshops. From time to time the trainer will have to be willing to submit to assessment.

Time to teach The trainer must be willing to make enough time available for teaching in the practice as well as for the associated activities in courses and workshops.

Clinical competence This is difficult for the selectors to assess. Factors which may be considered are:

The opinions of referees and committee members.
The possession of higher qualifications, especially the MRCGP.
The clinical records.

Good relationships with colleagues

Experience The trainer must have at least three years experience in general practice as a principal. This is a minimum period. It is not considered desirable for a trainer to be appointed after the age of sixty years.

Practice organisation The teaching practice must be well enough organised to facilitate teaching and to provide the necessary environment for learning how to run an efficient practice.

The records There must be in date order, and it is desirable that information is easily accessible for clinical and teaching purposes.

The premises These should provide adequate consultation rooms, office space and room for group discussions.

The equipment in the office and consultation room must be of a high standard.

Employed and attached staff must be seen to be functioning as an efficient team.

Appointment systems and duty rotas must be well organised. Full access to diagnostic facilities should be available.

The academic environment The teaching practice should provide the trainee with an environment which stimulates learning and encourages an inquiring state of mind. Audit activities should be a normal part of practice. There should be adequate books and journals in the practice library and there should be some evidence that they are used.

Cooperation Selection committees are expecting the whole practice to participate in teaching. All the partners should consider themselves as part of a teaching practice.

THE PROCESS OF SELECTION

1. Before you make any moves towards seeking selection, it is important that the whole practice thinks carefully about the

commitment it is taking on in terms of time and intellectual endeavour. Talk to the partners in other training practices and find out exactly what you are letting yourselves in for.
2. Once you are sure about your intentions, contact the local course organiser or the regional adviser in general practice. The secretary in the postgraduate centre you frequent will be able to give you their addresses.
3. The exact method of selection varies from region to region, but is likely to go through the following stages:
    a. You will have to attend a trainers' course during which you may be assessed for teaching ability and motivation.
    b. Your practice will be visited by an adviser who may be accompanied by other assessors from the LMC, the College or a trainers' workshop.
    c. The application is considered by the GP Education Committee. The power of selection is vested in the regional GP education committee or a visiting team of assessors. You and your practice will be assessed to see to what extent you fulfil the criteria for selection listed above. Do not be too depressed when you have read this list. Very few practices can meet all the criteria, and selection committees are reasonably pragmatic.

YOUR CONTINUING INVOLVEMENT

Once selected, you cannot sit back and rest on your laurels. You will be expected to:

* Participate in trainers workshops.
* Indulge in some postgraduate education activities.
* Keep your practice up to date.
* Show that you are actively seeking ways of improving your performance in patient care and teaching.

Medical politics

The majority of general practitioners ignore all aspects of medical politics and are often rather offhand about their colleagues who give up their time to represent them on various committees. It is important to realise just to what extent these political activities can affect the day-to-day work of the average general practitioner. If he or she wants better pay, better terms of service and better services for patients, then he or she must take an interest in medical politics. A GP may not feel inclined towards a career in medical politics, but at the least everyone should make sure that those who represent them hear their voice.

Below are a few notes on various medical organisations and how they may affect the GP.

LOCAL MEDICAL COMMITTEE

The local medical committee members are elected by the general practitoners. Each LMC covers the same area as the Family Practitioner Committee (FPC). The functions are:

* To collect and debate grassroots opinions about any aspect of medical politics. If a topic is considered to be of national importance, a motion can be put up to the annual conference of LMCs which is the policy-making body at national level.
* To arbitrate in disputes between colleagues.
* To make preliminary enquiries into complaints about GPs professional conduct.
* To investigate complaints by GPs about hospital services or any other problem that affect their work.
* To arbitrate in disputes with the FPC.

* To send representatives to other official committees which are concerned with general practice, e.g. the FPC, regional GP subcommittee, trainer selection committee.

An active and forward-thinking LMC can have a considerable influence on general practice at a local level, as well as influencing national policy-making.

THE DISTRICT HEALTH AUTHORITIES

The NHS reorganisation has given the DHAs considerable power to direct the development of patient services locally. As they provide all community health services, other than the GPs, changes in patterns of hospital care will always have an effect on the working conditions of local GPs. It is important for GPs to have a major influence on policy-making in the DHA.
DHA members are appointed by the Regional Health Authority from nominees put forward by a wide variety of political, voluntary and professional bodies.
The authority must have at least one GP and one consultant.
The DHA makes broad policy decisions but is not involved in day-to-day management.

The District Management Team has the real power! It is responsible for day-to-day management, as well as advising the DHA about policy.
The DMT should contain one GP and one consultant to represent the interests of their local colleagues. They should be nominated by the respective local bodies.
The DMT should be advised by a District Medical Committee, the members of which should be GPs and consultants in equal proportions. They should be elected. General practitioners must make sure that vigorous, pragmatic and forward-thinking colleagues are appointed to these organisations.

THE FAMILY PRACTITIONER COMMITTEE

The FPC is an independent body charged with the task of administering general practitioner, dental, ophthalmic and pharmaceutical services in the community. The GP is in contact with the FPC to provide a service for patients, and it has the responsibility of hearing complaints if the service obligations are not being met.

A friendly and cooperative FPC can do much to make life easier for GPs. Some of the members are nominees from the LMC, and it is important that they are the kind of people who can guide their colleagues on the committee to be sympathetic and realistic about the problems of general practice.

POSTGRADUATE EDUCATION

Postgraduate education is the responsibility of the Regional Postgraduate Dean, who is based in the appropriate university. Finance is provided by the university and by the regional hospital authority. Most of the money for general practitioner education comes from the DHSS. The dean's office administers the following officers and bodies:

1. Regional postgraduate education committee. Composed of representatives from all the medical disciplines. Makes broad policy decisions.
2. Regional general practice sub-committee. Members come from LMCs, the RCGP and undergraduate departments of GP. Responsible for administrating vocational training. More recently some have become involved in section 63 activities.
3. Regional GP advisers. University appointees who advise the GP sub-committee and implement its policies.
4. Clinical tutors. Appointed by the regional postgraduate committee to organise postgraduate activity at a local level. Usually consultants, but a few GP tutors are now being appointed on an experimental basis.

General practitioners can influence the style and content of their postgraduate educational activities by direct pressure on clinical tutors or by representations through their members on the GP sub-committee.

THE ROYAL COLLEGE OF GENERAL PRACTITIONERS

The RCGP is the academic voice of general practice. Founded in 1952, the membership is now in the region of 10000. It has functioned mainly as a 'think tank' for the evolution of practice and as a setter of standards.

* Membership is by examination which is held twice a year.
* Associate membership is also available and avoids the necessity of taking the examination.
* The RCGP publishes the college journal and issues frequent reports on various aspects of practice.
* Centrally, the council makes major policy decisions, organises some research and provides some educational activities.
* At a local level the Faculties arrange educational and organisational meetings. The principal value of these activities is to provide a forum for discussion and the generation of new ideas.
* The RCGP is concerned with the supervision of vocational training at a national level through the JCPT.

The College has considerable influence on the organisation of vocational and postgraduate education. The DHSS also appears to take careful note of the College's views when policy is being made.

Any GP who wants to be involved in determining the direction in which general practice will be steered in the future should consider joining the College and taking on active part in its deliberations.

Index

Accessibility, 64–70
    appointment system and, 64, 65–67
    covering out of hours, 69–70
    evening surgeries, 64–65
    home visits, 67–69
    practice nurse and, 65
Accountant, 136–137
Advertising, 134, 139
Age-sex register, 62, 102–103, 220–222
    computers and, 102–103, 231
    screening and, 56
Antenatal care, 49, 53, 59–60
    financial aspects, 132–133, 134
    practice protocol, 60, 237, 238–239
    record card, 60, 97
Appointment systems, 6, 65–67, 191–192
    receptionist and, 65
    urgent cases and, 66–67
Appropriate care, 22–22, 32–48
    chronic illness, 43–46
    investigation, 33–34
    minor illness, education and, 36–43
    prescribing, 34–36
    referral to hospital, 46–48
Audit, 103–107, 241–246
    clinical protocol formulation and, 106–107
    consultation analysis and, 104, 105
    mutual support and, 105–106
    prescribing and, 104, 242–244
    recall rate, 104, 242–244
    referral, 104–105, 245
    workload analysis and, 104
    workload management and, 122–123

Blood pressure screening, 53, 63, 97
    audit, 245
    records and, 209
Breast self examination, 51, 53, 59, 246

Call system, 108–109
Cervical smear, 51, 53, 59, 60, 62–63, 74
    age-sex register and, 102
    audit, 245, 246
    financial aspects, 132
    records and, 209
Chaperone, 110–111
Chemists, 182–183
Chronic illness, 8, 10, 43–46
    long-term surveillance by nurses, 125
    medical objectives and, 45–46
    recall system, 44–45
    regular visits, 44
    repeat prescriptions, 45
Clerical assistant, job description, 202–203
Clinic nurses, 175
Clinical assistant in hospital, 135
Comfort, 71–75, 108–118
Community midwives, 174–175
Computers, 45, 56, 102–103, 231–232
    age-sex register and, 102–103, 231
    accounting and, 102–103
    disease register and, 231
    morbidity register, 231
    recall register, 231
    records, 102–103, 232
    repeat prescribing and, 103, 231
    research and, 103
Confidentiality, 72, 75
Consultation
    audit, 104, 105
    call system, 108–109

equipment, 111
examining patients, 109–111
handling difficult people, 113–118
interruption by phone, 111–112
physical comfort and, 108–111
premises *see* Consulting room
psychological ease of doctor and, 111–118
speed, 112–113
technique *see* Consultant technique
Consultation length, 112
Consultation technique, 28–31, 247–249
analysis of recordings, 247–248
communication with patients, 29–31
consultation structure and, 248–249
explanation, 29, 30
formulating course of action, 29
information gathering, 28–29
information giving, 29, 30–31
minor illness and, 29–30
recording consultations, 249
taboo subjects and, 30
Consulting room, 108, 110
layout, 73, 109, 189–190
Contraceptive care, 51, 53, 59, 60
audit, 246
financial aspects, 131–132, 134, 135
records, 59, 209, 212
Convenience, 71–75
Cost, 74, 79–80
Country practice, 81–82

Delegation of work, 123–126, 129
district nurse and, 172
practice nurse and, 173–174
Deputising services, 70
Desk, doctor's, 73, 109, 289–290
Developmental surveillance, 52, 53–55
age-sex register and, 102
Diabetic nurse, 175, 176
Diagnosis, 29, 33
Diarrhoea, 42–43
Difficult patients, 113–118
iatrogenic aggression, 117–118
impact of serious illness, 116
manipulative patients, 115
psychopathic personalities, 116–117
rejection of responsibility, 114–116
Disabled people, 72, 188
Disease register, 231
District health authorities, 254
District nurses, 124–125, 140, 141, 150, 171–173

delegation and, 172
referral for procedures, 73
Doctor behaviour, 4, 8, 12, 13–15
competitiveness and, 14
workload and, 121–123

Effective service, 21
Efficient service, 21
Employment of staff, 156–159
contract of employment, 157
interviewing, 157
job description, 157
pay levels, 156, 158
selection of new staff, 156–157
training, 157–158
working conditions, 158–159
Ethics, 138, 139
Evening surgeries, 64–65
Examination, 109–111
chaperone and, 110–111
examination room, 110
Explanation, 29, 30, 40, 42

Facilities, practice, 34
Family practitioner committee, 254–255
Family responsibilities, 142–145
Fever, 41–42
Financial aspects, 12–13, 127–137
antenatal care, 132–133, 134
cervical smears, 132
claims for items-of-service, 129, 130, 133–134
contraception, 131–132, 134, 135
delegation and, 129
immunisation and, 130–131, 133–134, 135
informing patient of services and, 134–135
NHS fees, 130–135
private fees, 129–130, 135–136
spending priorities, 128–129
tax and, 136–137
Fringe practitioners, 181

Happiness, 19
Health education, 49–51
giving information, 50
see also Patient education
Health visitor, 61, 140, 141, 177–179
agreement of common policies, 178–179
partnership rules, 177–178

INDEX

role, 178
Home visits, 4, 6, 7, 67–69
  receptionist and, 68, 75
Hospital based community nurses, 175–176
Hospital doctors, 140
Hypertension, 97, 200
  see also Blood pressure screening

Immunisation, 51, 53, 60–61, 74, 223–226
  age-sex register and, 102
  children, 223
  financial aspects, 130–131, 133–134, 135
  follow-up babies, 223–225
  records and, 209
  travellers, 225–226
Income tax, 136–137
Information gathering, 28–29
Information giving, 29, 30–31, 35, 50
Interpractice relationships, 138–139
Intrapartum care, 174
Investigations, 33–34
  facilities, 73–74

Job description, 166, 202–206

Keeping up to date
  postgraduate education, 93–94
  practice literature, 93
  research and, 95
  Royal College of General Practitioners and, 95–96
  self-education, 92–94
  study leave, 94
  training activities and, 94–95

Local medical committee, 253–254

Measles, 199–200
Medical politics, 253–256
Meetings, workload management and, 122
Minor illness, 4, 8, 25, 32
  consultation technique and, 29–30
  diarrhoea/vomiting, 42–43
  education and, 36–43
  explanation and, 40
  self management, 32, 38, 39

upper respiratory tract infection, 40–42
Morbidity register, 231

National Health Service, 5–15
Nurses, 171–176

Obstetric list, 133
Optitian, 183
Otitis media, 40, 80, 123
Out of hours cover, 69–70
  deputising services and, 70
  GP rotas, 70
Outside interests, 143

Paramedical business people, 182–183
Partnership agreement, 90–91
Partnership relationships, 85–91
  delegation of organisation aspects, 88
  extrapractice committments and, 89, 90
  implementation of decisions, 87–88
  partnership agreement and, 90–91
  regular meetings and, 85–87
  sharing income, 88–90
  social interactions, 91
Patient education, 233–236
  minor illness and, 36–43
  patient information leaflet and, 234–236
  practice policy and, 233
Patient expectations, 4, 5, 12, 19–20
  workload and, 120–121
Patient information leaflet, 234–236
Personal care, 21, 23–31
  access to more than one doctor and, 23–24, 242
  care by practice, 24–25
  consultation technique and, 28–31
  minor illness and, 25–26
  problems in relating to patients and, 24–25
  reason for consultation and, 26–27
  tolerance/understanding and, 27–28
Post-graduate education, 93–94, 255
Postnatal care, 239–240
Practice diversity, 11–12
Practice literature, 93
Practice manager, 167–170
  accounting, 169
  administrative tasks, 169
  intrapractice communication and, 169–170

job description, 204–205
personnel management
supervision of routine systems, 168–169
teaching and, 170
Practice nurse, 13, 65, 124–125, 197–201
administrative aspects, 198–199
communications, 201
continuing education, 201
delegation, 173–174
direct employment, 173–174
immunisation and, 61
legal aspects, 201
medical/paramedial work, 198
nursing duties, 198
selection criteria, 199
training, 199–200
Practice organisation, 13
Practice premises, 188–190
see also Consulting room
Practice protocol, 83, 237–240
antenatal care, 60, 237, 238–239
audit, 106–107
chronic illness and, 46
preparation, 121, 237
prescribing and, 36
postnatal care, 239–240
Practice selection, 81–84
Prescribing, 34–36
audit, 104, 242–244
doctor's instructions and, 35
practice policy and, 36
see also Repeat prescribing systems
Prevention of disease, 49–63
health education, 49–51
records and, 209
screening, 51–63
Private income, 135–136
Private practitioners, 182
Psychiatric nurse, 175, 176

Reason for consultation, 26–27
Recall consultations, 121–123
audit, 104, 242–244
Recall system, 97
chronic illness, 44–45
computer and, 231
Reception area, 72
Receptionist, 13, 74–75, 116, 160–165
appointment system and, 65
home visits and, 68, 75
job description, 203–204
qualities required, 160–161
responsibilities, 163

support, 164–165
training, 161–163, 193–196
syllabus, 161–162
teaching sessions, 162–163
Recrods, 56, 96–103, 206–209
A4 record, 98, 207–208
age-sex register, 102
computers and, 102–103, 232
date order and, 98
file contents, 208–209
filing systems, 208
improvement of, 97–102
Lloyd-George envelope, 98, 207–208
planned care and, 97
prevention and, 209
recall system and, 97
recording consultation, 98, 209
special cards for long-term problems, 209–219
summarising, 100–101
Referral, 46–48
audit, 104–105, 245
referral letter, 47–48
Registering with a GP, 144–145
Repeat consultation *see* Recall consultation
Repeat prescribing system, 45, 75, 227–230
computers and, 103, 231
organisation, 227–230
record card, 212
Research, 95

computers and, 103
epidemiological, age-sex register and, 102
Rotas, out of hours cover and, 70
Royal College of General Practitioners, 95–96, 255–256
Rubella status, 51, 53, 61–62, 131
age-sex register and, 102
audit, 246

Screening, 51–63
age-sex register and, 56
criteria for procedure, 52
identifying patients, 56–58
organisation, 55–63
Secretary, 13, 166–167
job description, 204–205
Self-education, 92–94
Single-handed practices, 7, 11, 83
Size of practice list, 5, 6, 7
Social pathology, 10–11

Social workers, 140, 141, 180–181
Study leave, 94
Summary card, 100
Surgery accommodation, 158
Surgery site, 71–72

Team, practice, 149–183
   advantages, 153–154
   disadvantages, 154–155
   leadership, 152–153
   team versus network care, 151–152
Tolerance, 27–28
Tonsillitis, 40
Training practice, 94, 136, 250–252
   benefits of becoming, 250
   continuing involvement, 252
   requirements, 250–251
   selection, 251–252
Training staff, 157–158
   receptionists, 161–163, 193–196

Understanding, 27–28
Undertaker, 183
Upper respiratory tract infection, 40–42
Urban practice, 82

Verrucas, 235–236
Vomiting, 42–43

Waiting area, 72–73
Warts, 235–236
Workload, 7–11, 12
   audit, 104, 122–123
   delegation, 123–126
   doctor behaviour and, 121-123
   management, 119–126
   modification of patient expectations and, 120–121
   total hours worked, 119–120